Quality in the Veterans Health Administration

Quality in the Veterans Health Administration

Lessons from the People Who Changed the System

Galen L. Barbour

Larry Malby

Richard R. Lussier

R. W. Thomale Jr.

Judith A. Lerner

Editors

Foreword by Donald M. Berwick

Jossey-Bass Publishers • San Francisco

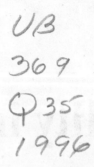

UB
369
Q35
1996

Substantial discounts on bulk quantities of Jossey-Bass books are available to corporations, professional associations, and other organizations. For details and discount information, contact the special sales department at Jossey-Bass Inc., Publishers (415) 433–1740; Fax (800) 605–2665.

For sales outside the United States, please contact your local Simon & Schuster International office.

 Manufactured in the United States of America on Lyons Falls Pathfinder Tradebook. This paper is acid-free and 100 percent totally chlorine-free.

Library of Congress Cataloging-in-Publication Data

Quality in the Veterans Health Administration : lessons from the
  people who changed the system / Galen L. Barbour . . . [et al.],
  editors ; foreword by Donald M. Berwick.
      p.   cm.
  Includes bibliographical references and index.
  ISBN 0-7879-0274-8 (alk. paper)
  1. United States. Veterans Health Administration—Management.
  2. Total quality management.   I. Barbour, Galen L., [date].
  [DNLM: 1. United States. Veterans Health Administration.
  2. Hospitals, Veterans—organization & administration—United
  States.   3. Total Quality Management.   UH 463 Q13 1996]
  UB369.Q35   1996
  362.1'0425—dc20
  DNLM/DLC
  for Library of Congress   96-2750
                                                                CIP

FIRST EDITION
HB Printing   10 9 8 7 6 5 4 3 2 1

Contents

Foreword

Like a luscious, ripe, bright red apple dangling from a tree, the fruit of "systemness" remains just beyond our grasp. We know what it would taste like, if we could reach it, but we stay hungry.

Our work creates a web of cause and effect. We are connected to each other. No matter how hard we struggle to define disciplines, departments, organizational boundaries, and local organizational cultures, we are inevitably and sometimes reluctantly bound together in the experiences we make for those who depend on us. Even when our work does not unite us, our purpose does— or it should.

We pay dearly for our divisions. Failing to act as a whole, we duplicate, drop, and deny. Our limits, which look so much to be from outside, lie, more than we can easily admit, within. We could do so much more with what we have, if only we could cooperate, if only we could act as a willing team, if only we could learn from each other and rely upon each other, if only we could embrace our commonalities with as much pride as we protect our differences.

We have learned so well to ask, "What am I made of?" and so poorly to inquire, "What am I part of?"

A sociologist from Mars, having studied the fragmentation of American health care generally, might turn to the Veterans Health Administration (VHA) with some excitement. "The rest are so divided," the Martian might say, "but here, at last, I'll bet there will be a difference." The Martian would see immediately how promising VHA is as a potential system. Look at its assets:

- *A common purpose.* "Without aim," said Dr. Deming, "there is no system." That is a fundamental insight, one that proposes, aims for, and *creates* a system. The elements of a system can be united by their common intent and, in the final analysis, by almost nothing else. In effect, the boundaries of a system are defined exactly by what the system is supposed to accomplish. If I were to define an intensive care unit (ICU) as "a place that maintains and improves physiological function in desperately ill people," you might not classify a hospital chaplain as part of an ICU. If I were to say that an ICU "treats the many needs of desperately ill people and their families," you might. Knowing aims helps to birth a system.

From this viewpoint, our Martian would notice that VHA is blessed with clarity. Its purpose is clear, largely because its customer base is well defined. Unlike most health care organizations, it was created for a very specific purpose. Score one point in favor of systemness.

- *A sense of being a team.* Just because there is a sense of purpose doesn't mean the people in the system know it. Often systemness runs aground because people do not feel involved in the aim. "Not," says the Martian, "in VHA, though." Look at the employees—doctors, nurses, technicians, managers, and other staff. From a purely objective standpoint, many would be better off elsewhere. The doctors could get paid more; the managers could have more authority. VHA scores low in mahogany and creature comforts, and to be frank, its share of patients with complex and frustrating needs is unusually large. There is a hint in all this that, perhaps, people work in VHA because they *want* to. They do feel that they are part of something larger than themselves. Score another point for systemness.

- *A strong infrastructure.* Systems need knitting. Much of health care suffers from its cottage industry thinking. Nothing binds the parts together; there is no fibrous tissue. So doctors work in their offices, distant from hospitals, with separate records, convinced of their distinctness. Hospitals are not nursing homes, nor do they share processes in common. Clinicians use *management* as a term of derision, while managers complain among themselves that physicians seem unhelpful. Doctors and nurses often write in separate sections of the medical record, and staunchly defend the separateness.

But VHA has fibrous tissue. Its people criticize their bureaucracy, but the Martian might well see its benefits, too. "These people complain about the central office," the Martian reports, "but they accept that they are in a relationship with it." As we read in this book by Barbour and many of his colleagues about VHA's journey toward improvement, those of us more familiar with the cottage industry marvel at forms of connection that the authors report almost offhandedly. VHA deploys training systems, holds video conferences, consolidates strategic plans, and, at least sometimes, makes decisions that echo everywhere throughout the system, while most of health care is still trying to tie its local shoelaces. The authors dutifully repeat the VHA mantra: "If you have seen one VHA hospital, you have seen one VHA hospital." It is a small joke made necessary by a larger reality: VHA is a connected whole, and one so powerful, I suspect, that the mantra is repeated in partial psychological defense against this knowledge of potentially overwhelming oneness. Score a third point for systemness.

• *A single payer.* Much of the health care industry is ripped apart by its payment structures—a monstrous collection of contradictory signals that Paul Batalden has called "the payment system from hell." In the hospital that must shorten its lengths of stay to gain contracts from managed care systems that are making risk contracts with doctors, those same doctors may be getting paid more for longer stays for fee-for-service patients. The same multispecialty clinic whose new health maintenance organization is fighting to keep ancillary testing costs down may make a large profit on X-rays for its indemnity-insured patients. Crazy payment begets crazy behavior.

"Aha!" cries the Martian, "good sense at last." VHA has what it takes to make finance and systemness align: it has a single budget. The internal squabbles are inevitable, but when the day is done, the money comes from all one pot, and robbing Peter to pay Paul means Paul pays Peter too. I admit to my own devotion to a single-payer mechanism as the only sensible approach to health care finance I can think of. I also admit that neither I nor my grandchildren will likely see that in the United States before we are senile. But, like the Martian, I see islands of potential financial sanity, and VHA is one. It is, of course, under financial pressure; that is because it is in the real world. But, because of its budgeting form, it ought to be able to see finance, like its work, as part of a system of the whole. Waste reduction, for example, if properly managed, should return real benefits to VHA, supporting its purpose and sustainability. In much of the health care industry, by contrast, such efforts simply mean that one person yields profits to another. Score another point for systemness.

The Martian could go on to notice other conditions in VHA that are favorable to systemness: its potential for a unified information system; its public-domain quality, which permits (even requires) the open spread of news; its shared pride in its history of successful research and development; and its commitment to building the management capabilities of its leaders.

And so, as we pick up this book recounting the story of VHA's efforts to develop a system for total quality improvement (TQI), we, like the Martian, expect a complete success story—perhaps even the Holy Grail of what we all could be, if only we had the special qualities that allow VHA to be what we all should be: a system of the whole. Alas, this book does not provide a final, complete model for system improvement. Rather, we find here the difficult struggle that we, pursuers of improvement, all are going through. We find here not a model but a mirror, as the authors lead us through a journey fraught with persistent struggle as inexorable as Matthew Arnold's description of the ocean waves that "draw back and fling, / At their return, up the high strand, / Begin, and cease, and then again begin." In complete candor, the authors tell us at the outset that they have not yet grasped the apple of systemness. "Why?" asks the Martian. "What's wrong?"

And then, with somewhat mixed feelings, we find that the authors never intended to claim discovery of the Grail. Their story is confined to the formative years of 1992 to 1994, when VHA set out to implement a system of improvement. In their words, "This story is about learning to walk." Our Martian was looking for the apple of systemness in a book about planting an apple tree. And a fascinating story it is. We see faults, even failures; we experience the competing forces inherent in any system; we are allowed to question strategy along with the authors; we see how a system tends to shape issues in the face of massive investment and planning that tries to dictate otherwise.

The authors could have told a different story. This book *is* filled with many successes. VHA has developed a superb-quality training system. It has set out to make good use of procedures for organizational self-assessment based on Baldrige criteria. In a few areas, it has successfully focused its own collaborative energies on important clinical topics like cardiac care and certain problems in rehabilitation. Undoubtedly, Barbour and his colleagues were sorely tempted to focus on such successes. Chapter Twelve, for example, recounts a series of early team success stories, delightfully expressed in the vernacular of actual team members. It is a chapter that stands like an island, as if to reassure the reader that VHA did experience much success: TQI teams reduced bed cleaning times by half, shortened warehouse-to-pharmacy drug delivery times by more than 90 percent, and dramatically increased the immunization rate of high-risk outpatients in just one year. Such team activities represent hundreds of successful outcomes, yet the authors resisted the temptation to make this a book of local success stories. They remained faithful to their systemic view.

The authors also resisted reaching past their intended time frame of 1992 to 1994. Had they done so, they could point to a significant increase in the average VHA hospital accreditation scores from the Joint Commission on Accreditation of Healthcare Organizations (JCAHO) in 1995. JCAHO's agenda for change looks for implementation of many of the principles embodied in TQI, and these higher scores are likely evidence of the effect of TQI implementation in the VHA system. Perhaps we can score another point for systemness. The authors also could have pointed to sweeping organizational changes made in 1995 and 1996 under the new leadership of Ken Kizer, who succeeded Jim Holsinger as undersecretary for health, changes that were designed to allow VHA to take better advantage of its system strengths. These are the stuff of a book yet to be written.

For those tempted to wait for the sequel, I would counsel, "Reader, find here an image of yourself." Study the assets that made—and *still* make—VHA one of the most promising of all of America's health care systems when it comes to fundamental system improvement. And then learn here in distilled form about the barriers that formed despite that promise. Keep asking why, with a clear mission, a strong sense of belonging, a single payer, a well-developed managerial infrastructure, and other strengths, the story that Barbour and his colleagues tell us about VHA is so vaguely familiar to our own experiences.

How the story ultimately plays out remains to be seen. An old maxim says, "One who does not learn from the past is bound to repeat it." Hidden between the lines of the story told here are the decelerators that are so regular and recurrent in early efforts toward system improvement. VHA would do well not to repeat them.

1. *Senior leadership inattention.* There is a long distance between senior executive *permission* to manage quality and senior executive *direction* of the improvement process. We read in this book how Jim Holsinger was prevented from directing the TQI rollout by an action filed by the American Federation of Government Employees Union, which charged VHA officials with an unfair labor practice. Although that proscription was lifted by an agreement reached in 1994, the forced removal of direct involvement by top leadership made their participation look simply like permission. Even the best executives have to learn the difference between permission and direction through experience. What they learn is this: improvement cannot be merely permitted; it must be driven by the day-to-day attention of top leaders and evidenced in their activities in review, clarification, teaching, celebration, and personal application.

2. *Programmatic thinking.* In the early stages, almost all organizations try to make quality improvement a "program." It falls onto a list of desired activities and is assigned to staff. In the short run, much action follows. In the longer run, that action fails to meet the organization's fundamental need to improve. The problem lies in splitting the quality improvement effort from the organization's core work and strategies. I sometimes wish there were no word, *quality,* to seduce us into the reductionist view of improvement as a "program." What "part" of a child learns to walk? The question is silly. For exactly the same reasons, we cannot meaningfully ask what part of a system creates quality.

3. *Failure to link quality improvement to strategy.* In its mature forms, quality improvement is a survival strategy. When this is true in an organization, if you ask an executive, "How will you thrive?" the answer will be, "By getting better at everything we do." An organization is not yet there when it still talks about quality and cost as separate topics. (You can also tell whether quality is understood as strategy by examining the minutes of board meetings.)

4. *Staying stuck in theory.* Quality improvement must become the domain of the actual work of the organization, not just a methodology. Improvement is a physical thing. A thousand Pareto analyses amount to nothing at all unless work changes. Partly because of overdelegation to staff (see Decelerator 1) and partly because of lack of confidence in improvement as a strategy (see Decelerator 3), quality improvement efforts often become too focused on methods and models and avoid making changes and learning inductively from them. If you wish to predict how fast an organization is likely to improve, don't count its retreats or quality improvement training classes, count the number of changes it is testing in its actual work processes.

Not being in VHA, I cannot be sure which, if any, of these decelerators are now standing in their way. Nor can I gainsay the extraordinary scale of the efforts that Barbour and his colleagues describe. It is a story that exists nowhere else. They have much to be proud of. By writing this book with such a clear sense of purpose, they not only let us celebrate with them what they have done so far but also invite us to reflect with genuine curiosity on what now could happen to help them go even farther and faster in the pursuit of systemic improvement. I suspect that our Martian, intrigued by this description of the early struggles of a system in change, may already be planning a return trip to see how VHA, a system with so much promise, comes out. Perhaps by that time, that tree planted in the early 1990s will be bearing fruit, and some of it may have grown within reach.

June 1996   Donald M. Berwick
                                    Institute for Healthcare Improvement
                                    Boston, Massachusetts

Preface

This book tells the story of how the Department of Veterans Affairs (VA) made a commitment to change and turned that commitment into a transformation of its hospitals, its health care delivery system, and its people. Senior management at VA decided to endorse the precepts of total quality management (TQM)—renaming it total quality improvement (TQI)—as the proper vehicle for making that transformation. There was enthusiasm for widespread change at the very beginning, but when the department's plan began to develop cracks and threatened to crumble, the strength of its commitment was severely tested. It lasted, however, and a new plan for change was crafted and instituted. There were successes and there were problems and failures, but we learned from each one and tried to use that new knowledge to improve the implementation process.

Our intention in this book is to convey the aim of the original plan and the rationale for settling on that particular implementation scheme. We will also describe the problems that arose, the intrinsic barriers we encountered, and the places where we stumbled. This book is unique because it provides information about the implementation of TQM in a nationwide, government-run hospital system. The national scope of the Veterans Health Administration's project made it substantially different from other TQM implementations. But since VA encountered virtually every type of legal and regulatory barrier and substantial political pressure—both positive and negative—along the way, its experience is useful for anyone trying to change the health care culture to TQM, no matter the venue. There are lessons about the process at both the hospital and the system level.

The foothold of TQM in the United States is now steadily growing. In 1990, when VA endorsed the concept for its health care system (renaming it TQI due to concern on the part of some employees

over the term *management*), it was just becoming recognized as
a valuable management tool in the manufacturing and industrial
sectors of our economy. At that time, experience with putting
the principles and precepts of TQM into practice in the service
industry—let alone the health care industry—was scant and published accounts of it even scantier. What was appearing in the
medical literature of the time were stories about single departments or divisions that had applied TQM ideas to issues in their
practice. There was not much published about experiences with
TQM in entire hospitals. Berwick, Godfrey, and Roessner's *Curing
Health Care* (1990) reported on the findings of the National
Demonstration Project, which began in 1987; in 1990 Marszalek-
Gaucher and Coffey wrote *Transforming Healthcare Organizations,* an
account of their experience with the University of Michigan Hospitals. These two signal works provided the evidence that TQM
could be successfully implemented in health care settings.

The Department of Veterans Affairs health care system—
managed by the Veterans Health Administration (VHA)—is a
large, highly integrated system of hospitals, clinics, and nursing
homes spread all across America. There is a VHA presence in every
state. The system provides a sizeable part of the health care delivered in the country every year: it treats approximately one million
inpatients and twenty-four million outpatients annually. It provides
all types of care, even organ transplants. For a period of some
years, the quality of the health care delivered by VHA was questioned by lawmakers and the media, based on anecdotal cases with
less-than-optimum outcomes. By the late 1980s, VHA had made
several attempts to correct identified deficiencies by traditional
means—quality assurance evaluations and headquarters pronouncements about needed changes. These proved ineffective, however.
Something different was needed for VHA to demonstrate the quality of care it provided and to identify and improve those areas where
outcomes were unacceptable. But like the rest of U.S. government
at the end of the 1980s, the Department of Veterans Affairs was facing budgetary cutbacks, and it appeared likely that VHA would once
again simply be admonished to "do more with less."

In August 1990, the secretary of veterans affairs, Edward Derwinski,
selected a new chief medical director to head VHA and deal with
quality concerns and the tight budget. The new director was James
W. Holsinger Jr., M.D., a veteran himself and a longtime employee

of Veterans Affairs. Holsinger had served as both chief of staff and director of a VA hospital during his tenure, and he brought with him a clear understanding of the problems and the culture of VHA. As he stepped into the job of being VHA's highest-ranking physician, Holsinger brought with him several new faces to VHA headquarters. He completely reorganized VHA's central office and accountability structure and even created some new functions at VHA's top levels. One such function was quality assurance oversight. Previously located three tiers lower, this office now reported directly to the chief medical director.

One of Holsinger's key intentions as he entered office was to address VHA's culture and the quality of its services by instituting TQI throughout the entire system. The man he chose to lead this endeavor was John Fears, himself a former hospital director at several VA facilities. Fears had successfully instituted TQI practices the preceding year at the Hines VA hospital in Chicago. The time was ripe for change: the face of health care administration was in flux across the country, without a clear direction or target, and national health care reform was looming on the horizon as the cost of health care in all settings continued to grow rapidly, in spite of attempts by insurers and employers to curb the escalation. Obviously, the old solutions were not working, and something more dramatic was needed—a perception shared by many of the hospital directors across the VHA system. As they faced increased demand for services, rising costs of care, and a shrinking budget, these men and women were also searching for a meaningful way to maintain and improve quality. Many of them turned to TQM; some had engaged consultants to assist them in becoming aware of the process even before 1990.

Under the guidance of Jim Holsinger, those of us in VHA's central office and the majority of the system's hospital directors undertook the enormous challenge of bringing TQI practices and precepts to a huge bureaucratic system of health care. We began in 1991 after a year of planning and organizing and after contracting with a national consultant to assist in the process. A thorough presentation of TQI to the entire system was not completed until 1995, and the need for support, resource distribution, and training still continues. Also, at the time we began to make our first plans and develop our training programs, there was little in the literature about TQM in hospitals and even less about implementing TQM across an entire health care system. Probably the largest system that had attempted such an endeavor was Hospital Corporation of America in Nashville, Tennessee, under the guidance of Paul Batalden and Eugene Nelson, whose efforts provided the only glimpse of what we might be facing. But VHA could not wait for others to plow that ground. We began our own implementation effort, and this book tells the story of what happened.

Audience

This book is written primarily for all leaders and managers of health care systems and hospitals, public and private. From the chief executive officer of a large hospital chain to the board members of a multihospital system or the executives, physicians, managers, and supervisors in an individual hospital, the lessons in VHA's experience are pertinent and of practical value. We present the information in a manner that will be helpful to all employees— each one can learn about his or her role in the necessary transformation by studying our experiences and coming to understand the interrelationship of all roles in producing continuous improvement in health care. Those in top management can benefit from our experience by noting the type of organizational planning and follow-through we pursued from the upper reaches of the organization to ensure success. Physicians, nurses, and other practitioners whose primary focus is the individual hospital where they work can also find important lessons in this book regarding the importance of involving all employees, providing appropriate education and feedback, and supporting their local quality improvement teams in their activities.

The secondary audience for this book consists of two segments of government employees. The first are those employees who would like information and encouragement to help them and their fellow employees know and believe that continuous improvement is not impossible in government. It is difficult, but it is not impossible. These are the individuals who will be responsible for achieving TQI changes and improvements; this book will make them aware of the support they should expect, support that is necessary for their success. The second group are those involved in the oversight and funding of government operations; they need examples of how federal organizations can be encouraged to develop a TQI culture without the threat of budget reductions. The public sector has the capability to implement the principles of continuous improvement, but it will take time and some degree of front-loading. These lessons, and the clear advantages of TQI to the government and the taxpayer, are evident in this book.

The lessons and experiences described in this book are also of value to private sector health care organizations and professionals, including health maintenance organizations, insurers, suppliers, professional societies and organizations, accrediting agencies, academic institutions, employers, managers, and management trainees. Students of health care administration, consultants in health care management, and researchers in the fields of performance improvement and organizational development also may benefit from reading this book; although the lessons are drawn from a vast government health care system, they have meaning and pertinence for all health care settings.

Overview of the Contents

The book is presented in four parts. The first two chapters in Part One introduce the challenges facing VHA, the history of federally supported health care for the nation's veterans, and the role VHA has come to play in American health care. The structure and culture of the VHA system is presented so the reader will understand the need for change and the unique difficulties faced by VHA in pursuing it. Chapter Three presents a rapid overview of the history of TQM, describing its acceptance by industry, the development of the Malcolm Baldrige Award, and some early total quality efforts in health care. The chapter lays an important foundation for Part Two, which bridges the discussions of the industrial and health care models of TQI and covers the early phases of VHA's involvement. Chapter Four focuses on the actions and impact of VHA leaders who began to endorse, teach, and practice continuous improvement in some of our hospitals well in advance of the 1991 national implementation program. These pioneers helped develop positive attitudes and experiences in key parts of the organization, and the authors argue that these early efforts helped prepare the system for the national rollout that began in 1991. Chapter Five describes the implementation of TQI at the Hines VA hospital and pays particular attention to important developments at VHA's central office that inspired crucial support for TQI when Jim Holsinger and John Fears started planning for it in 1990. Chapter Six presents the rationale behind VHA's decision to pursue TQI and examines its plan for systemwide implementation: develop teaching methods at a small number of hospitals, collect feedback on the efficacy of those methods, and make any necessary changes in the process before moving on to a larger number of hospitals to repeat the process. The plan called for four implementation phases, each taking about one year; an important part of the plan was to gradually move responsibility for TQI training and support away from outside consultants and toward newly trained VHA personnel. The intent of this part of the plan was to save VHA a sizable amount of money, which could then be used to support the rollout process over the four-year implementation period.

Part Three covers important aspects of the actual implementation of TQI in a large federal bureaucracy. Chapters Seven through Nine form a trilogy on the issue of leadership, discussing the roles of physician leaders, senior executives, and mid-level managers, respectively. Chapter Seven addresses one of the most critical issues for health care organizations implementing TQI: involving physicians in the implementation process. VHA's physicians are full-time employees of the department; therefore, enlisting their support presented different challenges than enlisting the support of physicians in a private hospital. Part of VHA's plan, detailed in this chapter, was to develop a trained cadre of internal physician consultants who would visit each new facility during its implementation effort and directly address the local physicians about their involvement. This emphasis on recruitment of local physician support was an important part of the success of the overall implementation. Chapter Eight, written by an internal TQI physician consultant, examines the importance of involving the top leadership in individual hospitals. Although the critical nature of top management's support is well known, some of the information presented here underscores that importance with new information about the impact of stable leadership. Chapter Nine contrasts the emphasis placed on physicians in implementing TQI in health care organizations with the general lack of attention paid to an equally important segment of the workforce—the mid-level managers and supervisors. The chapter presents several important lessons about how these key individuals should be brought into the process and what will happen to the best-laid TQI plans if these employees aren't involved. Chapter Ten recounts the successes and difficulties encountered by VA hospitals in performing organizational assessments. As this chapter demonstrates, for large systems it is important to use the same approach and assessment instruments at each facility. On the other hand, the chapter also stresses the importance of using institutional memory and judgment to mold the assessment *process* to each individual site, and it presents a number of ways to do this. Chapter Eleven focuses on the critical importance of training, for all levels of employees. The chapter recounts the emphasis on training in VHA's plan and describes how the needs of individual sites were met using a centralized approach and TQI "master trainers." This part of the implementation was clearly the most costly, but it could not have been slighted without creating the potential for serious problems in the future.

Part Four details the results of the implementation process and relates specific outcomes. These chapters reflect upon the implementation process primarily from the perspective of the hospital, although they briefly orient the reader to the systemwide view as well in order to illustrate the connection between local activities and the overall plan. Chapter Twelve presents a series of vignettes describing TQI experiences from the early phase of the implementation, told by the actual practitioners involved. Chapter Thirteen covers the overall experience VHA had with the use of TQI's key tool—the team. Team dynamics, training, chartering, and support are explained and dissected to obtain a number of important lessons and alert the reader to potential pitfalls.

Chapters Fourteen and Fifteen address the TQI rollout from a wider perspective. In Chapter Fourteen, the authors discuss the rollout from the perspective of one of VHA's four regions, providing important insights into the time and resource requirements of a successful implementation. In Chapter Fifteen, the authors look at the implementation of continuous improvement principles from the perspective of the VHA system as a whole. They review the major lessons learned at that level from the master trainers and VHA's centralized support functions, examining both local and global activity. With the recognition that the implementation plan had been overcome by events, serious rethinking was done in preparation for the continuation of the rollout after the first thirty-eight hospitals were engaged. Chapter Sixteen depicts the new plan and sets the stage for the report of the rollout to the remaining 140 VA hospitals that occurred in 1994.

Each of the chapters was written by experienced individuals with deep involvement in the plan and the implementation process. All prepared their submissions, by request, for this book; their opinions and contributions do not constitute a consensus, and they contain some degree of overlap and repetition. We have allowed this to remain since it underscores important points and issues from differing perspectives.

Acknowledgments

I wish to thank a number of people for their time and efforts in support of this book. First, there are those who made this book possible by virtue of who they were and what they did in the larger scheme of VHA's implementation of TQI. Foremost is Robert Cullen, Ph.D., a man of great compassion and strong determination who steered the TQI rollout unerringly through many troublesome times as chair of the VHA TQI coordinating committee. The task of coordinating the massive TQI training effort fell to the staff of the TQI education and support division at the St. Louis continuing education center (CEC). Under Lynn Ward's leadership, the CEC staff of Ann Strong, Janet Reese, Linda White, and Brenda Bowder provided "just-in-time" encouragement, support, and funding for the critical training needs of the hospitals. That small group in the Office of Resource Management who charted the beginnings in the VHA central office headquarters—Patricia Hicks, Marianne McGuire, and Carol Arndt—deserve special mention and praise. I am particularly grateful to the American Productivity and Quality Center (APQC) Consulting Group, who provided early guidance, support, and continuous consulting services, and especially Lyell Jennings, Paul Murphy, Jerry Fuller, Susan Siferd, and Patricia Shockley for their tireless efforts in helping VHA initiate the TQI program. In particular, I want to thank all those who made this book possible through identifying necessary sources and providing us material and information for the chapters. VHA master trainers who contributed their knowledge and insight during lengthy structured interviews were Adrienne Fenev, Kurt Gundacker, Karen McCoy, Marisa Palkuti, Debra Peeples, and Kolman Rosenberg. A special thanks also goes to Jeff Bellah and Bob Krause, executive assistants for TQI who went out of their way to make unique contributions and to help me fill in gaps in my knowledge and in the manuscript. Morgan Bantley and Dale Turner of VHA's National Media Center contributed the artwork for the book. A special tribute must go to Fred Malphurs, Mary Ellen Piché, and the entire staff of the Albany VA medical center for helping show the way to TQI and for being the first-ever recipient in VHA of the coveted Robert W. Carey Award. It is always unfortunate that those we count on the most are too numerous to mention; in this case, VHA's TQI journey would never have succeeded had it not been for the tireless work of the hundreds of executive assistants for TQI and quality managers who really brought "continuous improvement" to light and whose stories are the very fabric of this book. There should be a special mention for Richard Lussier, whose vision and early nurturing as head of the TQI publications committee carried this book forward. And finally, I want to thank all the spouses and friends of the editors and authors for their support, especially my wife, Carolyn Barbour, and Larry Malby's wife, Virginia Malby, who put up with the long hours and many disruptions to family schedules needed to complete this book. Without their active encouragement and support we would not have been able to finish the work.

This book is dedicated to one who made it possible, Jim Holsinger, and to some who remind us what VHA is all about, Marine Lieutenants Gatlin "Jerry" Howell, Ivars Lama, Glen McCarty, and Larry Stone, whose faces are indelibly inscribed in memory and whose names are forever enshrined on "the wall" at the Vietnam Veterans Memorial.

June 1996   Galen L. Barbour
                                                  Washington, D.C.

References

Berwick, D. M., Godfrey, A. B., & Roessner, J. (1990). *Curing health care: New strategies for quality improvement.* San Francisco: Jossey-Bass.

Marszalek-Gaucher, E., & Coffey, R. J. (1990). *Transforming healthcare organizations.* San Francisco: Jossey-Bass.

The Editors

Senior Editor

Galen L. Barbour is the director of planning, education, and performance improvement at the Washington, D.C., VA medical center. Between August 1990 and September 1995 he served as the associate chief medical director for quality management for the Veterans Health Administration (VHA) and was responsible for designing, developing, and overseeing various quality assessment and improvement programs for VHA's 172 hospitals and all of its clinics and nursing homes throughout the country. Since 1990 he has held a position as a clinical professor in the Department of Internal Medicine at The George Washington University School of Medicine.

He has held positions of increasing administrative responsibility over a thirty-year career in the Department of Veterans Affairs, including director of the dialysis unit at the VA hospital in Little Rock, Arkansas; chief of the medical service at the VA hospital in Hampton, Virginia; and professor and vice-chairman of the Department of Internal Medicine at the Medical College of Hampton Roads. He became associate chief medical director of VHA in 1990.

His most recent efforts have been in the area of creating tools to measure the quality of health care and in the development of a balanced set of measures to reflect the quality of care in the VHA system. He has published numerous articles in the fields of nephrology, internal medicine, quality assurance, and performance improvement and has lectured nationally about VHA's programs and measurement capabilities. He has served as a consultant to medical societies and academic organizations in Switzerland and Turkey and to the Department of Defense's Uniformed Services University of the Health Sciences. He is currently a reviewer for several medical journals.

Coeditors

Larry Malby is the national total quality improvement (TQI) coordinator for the Veterans Health Administration. Since 1991 he has administered the rollout of the TQI process throughout VHA. He is a Marine Corps veteran of the Vietnam War and has served in a variety of positions in his twenty-three years of VHA service, including clinical social worker, internal auditor, systems planner, and correspondence analyst. He earned master's degrees in education, from the University of Idaho (1971), and social work, from the University of Washington (1973), under the auspices of the vocational rehabilitation program run by the Department of Veterans Affairs.

Richard R. Lussier is deputy director at VHA's Long Beach regional medical education center. He received a baccalaureate degree from California State University, Long Beach (1967), in health science and a doctor of public health degree from UCLA (1970). Following graduation, Dr. Lussier taught for five years at UCLA and for twenty-one years at California State University, Long Beach. During his tenure at California State University, he served as the coordinator of undergraduate education in health science, director of graduate studies, department chair, and director of a research institute. Dr. Lussier has extensive consulting experience in the areas of strategic planning and organizational transitions in the private and public sectors.

R. W. Thomale Jr. is the chief of acquisitions and materiel management at the Dallas VA medical center. He has served as a TQI coordinator and as an instructor for various courses, including TQI. He received a B.S. degree in education (1969) from Concordia Teachers College in Seward, Nebraska.

Judith A. Lerner is a program manager at VHA's Long Beach regional medical education center. She received a baccalaureate degree in mathematics from Miami University (1971) and a master's degree in adult and continuing education from the University of Illinois (1979). Following graduation, Ms. Lerner joined the staff of the Long Beach regional medical education center and has served there in many capacities. She has extensive experience in teaching, educational and instructional design, and organizational consulting on strategic planning and organizational transitions, both inside and outside the health care setting.

The Contributors

Kenneth J. Clark is the director of the VA medical center in West Los Angeles, California. He received a B.S. degree (1972) from Ithaca College, an M.H.A. degree (1975) from George Washington University, and a J.D. degree (1982) from Loyola Law School.

Linda C. Exner is a career employee with VHA. She currently holds the position of acting associate director of VHA's Durham, North Carolina, regional medical education center. Ms. Exner received a B.S.N. (1970) and M.S.N. (1979) from the Duke University School of Nursing, where she also holds a consulting faculty appointment. She has been involved with VHA's TQI efforts since 1991 as both a master trainer and consultant.

John R. Fears is currently director of the Carl T. Hayden VA hospital in Phoenix, Arizona. He has held numerous senior positions within the VHA health care system, including the position responsible for budgeting and planning for all medical facilities in the system. He received a B.S. degree (1963) from the University of South Carolina and a J.D. (1967) from the University of Oklahoma.

Kenneth D. Flint is a health care education officer and certified TQI educator/consultant for VHA. He works as a consultant in the national TQI implementation effort at various VHA medical facilities. As program manager at the Long Beach regional medical education center, he designs, implements, and evaluates education programs for health care professionals. He completed his undergraduate work in international relations and Latin American studies at the University of California at Los Angeles (1967). His graduate work includes a master's degree in political science from California State University at Long Beach (1974) and completion of a certificate program from the Nonprofit Management Institute of the University of California at Irvine.

Stuart C. Gilman is director of the Long Beach regional medical education center. He received an M.D. degree from Rush Medical College, Chicago (1983), and an M.P.H. from the University of California at Los Angeles (1989). Gilman was a VA/Robert Wood Johnson scholar at the University of California at San Francisco (1989). He is currently clinical assistant professor of medicine at the University of California at Irvine.

John C. Lammers is a former health system specialist with VHA's Western Region Special Studies Group. He currently is an assistant professor in the Department of Communication at the University of California at Santa Barbara and an adjunct assistant professor in the school of public health at the University of California at Los Angeles. He received M.S. (1980) and Ph.D. (1985) degrees in sociology from the University of California at Davis.

David K. Lee is clinical associate professor of medicine at the University of Washington and chief of staff at the Boise, Idaho, VA hospital. He received a B.A. degree (1969) from Johns Hopkins University and an M.D. degree (1973) from Harvard Medical School.

M. Jo MacDonald is the director of VHA's Quality Management Institute and Education Center in Durham, North Carolina. Ms. MacDonald has worked at VHA facilities in Northport, New York; West Los Angeles, California; and Durham since 1981, with roles in vocational rehabilitation, quality management, and continuing medical education. She received a B.A. degree (1966) in Christian education from West Virginia Wesleyan College and an M.S. in education (1981) from Hofstra University. She received her Ed.D. degree (1996) in adult and community college education at North Carolina State University and is a certified professional in health care quality.

Evereteen Mayfield is the acting chief of social work at the VA hospital in Dallas, Texas, where she is also the TQI coordinator for the social work service. She received a B.A. degree (1969) in sociology from LeMoyne-Owen College and an M.S.W. degree (1971) from the University of Michigan.

Robert P. Means is deputy director of VHA's regional medical education center in Cleveland, Ohio. He received a B.A. degree (1969) in political science and history from Drake University and an M.Ed. (1974) in higher education administration and a Ph.D. (1979) in adult and continuing education from the University of Illinois at Champaign-Urbana.

Gene D. Mickelson has ten years' experience as an education program and training consultant focusing on mid-level and senior management training and education. He has been involved in the design and implementation of numerous education programs and workshops in the areas of strategic planning, organizational change, assessment of leadership styles, effective communication, and team building. For the past four years he has served as a TQI master trainer assisting organizations in assessing, diagnosing, and implementing strategies for improving processes and overall performance. Prior to joining the Minneapolis regional medical education center, Mickelson was executive director for a physician professional standards review organization located in southern Minnesota. He also has had experience as a hospital administrator.

John P. Morrison is the TQI coordinator at the VA hospital in Oklahoma City. He received a B.S. degree (1979) from Middle Tennessee State University and an M.P.H. degree (1991) from the University of Oklahoma.

Joseph R. Nagel is associate director of VHA's regional medical education center in Cleveland, Ohio. He received a B.A. degree (1970) in sociology from Cleveland State University, an M.A. degree (1976) in community health education from Kent State University, and an Ed.D. degree (1986) in higher education administration from the University of Akron.

Steven R. Orwig is an assistant professor at Oklahoma State College of Medicine and is associate chief of staff for education at the Oklahoma City VA hospital, where he has served on the TQI steering committee since its creation in 1991. He is also a member of the national VHA TQI coordinating committee. He attended Austin College and Texas Tech University as an undergraduate and received an M.D. degree (1979) at the University of Texas Medical School at San Antonio.

Kathryn K. St. Morris is the chief of the quality management service and a TQI master trainer at the San Diego VA hospital. She has served as executive assistant to the director for TQI, associate chief of the nursing service, and in many other nursing roles, including as a nursing instructor in Honduras with the Peace Corps. She received a B.S.N. (1978) from the University of California, San Francisco, and an M.S.N. (1988) in nursing administration from San Diego State University.

Jack R. Sklar is the quality improvement coordinator at the Long Beach VA medical center. He is the former TQI team leader from the Long Beach regional medical education center. He received a B.A. degree from California State University, Long Beach (1973) in physical education and corrective therapy. He is also a certified kinesiotherapist.

Sherry Treiber is the total quality coordinator of the Western Pennsylvania network of VA hospitals, where she provides consultation and support services for a full range of organizational change and improvement efforts. She also participates in a variety of national initiatives relating to planning, training, and coordinating current and future directions for VHA. She received a B.S. degree (1979) in nursing and an M.S. degree (1990) in psychiatric/mental health nursing from Arizona State University.

Lynn D. Ward is the director of the TQI Education and Support Division located at VHA's St. Louis continuing education center. Prior to assuming the TQI position, Dr. Ward conducted local, regional, and national training programs in quality assurance and management development. She has worked for VHA for fifteen years and has clinical and administrative experience in nursing and as an assistant professor of nursing at Southern Illinois University at Edwardsville. She received B.S.N. (1966) and M.S.N. (1974) degrees and a doctorate in education (1987) from Southern Illinois University at Edwardsville.

Quality in the Veterans Health Administration

In 1990, during the six months after President George Bush had appointed me chief medical director of the Department of Veterans Affairs but prior to my confirmation by the Senate, I had the opportunity to carefully consider a variety of issues facing the Veterans Health Administration (VHA). Recognizing that a new team would have an opportunity to rapidly make a difference, I pondered where we could make the greatest difference in the shortest period of time.

A key issue facing me and the new team of leaders who had agreed to come to Washington with me was the quality of veterans' health care; questions had been raised about this issue by several observers, and this seemed a clear target of opportunity. Since total quality management (TQM) techniques had been found to make a difference in a variety of industries, there seemed no reason they would not work in a large, dispersed organization like VHA.

I believed there would be no better time to develop radically new ways of dealing with quality issues than at the time a new team began to lead VHA. We clearly had the opportunity to use new approaches to deal with time-worn problems. TQM, I believed, could and would make that difference. TQM techniques empower people at all levels of an organization to make a difference, and if ever an organization needed all the brain power it could muster, it was VHA in the fall of 1990. I wanted new and liberating methods to deal with the issues facing us, and I felt TQM could give us the edge and catapult VHA out of a slough of despondency and into a new era of sustained quality. And I felt we had the right people to do just that.

Lexington, Kentucky   James W. Holsinger Jr.
June 1996

Part One

The Seeds of Change

Chapter One

Learning to Ask the Right Questions

Galen L. Barbour

Health care delivered by the Department of Veterans Affairs, or VA (formerly the Veterans Administration), has been a major component of American medicine for decades. The more than 170 VA medical centers, consistently organized along lines of vertically integrated health care delivery, include outpatient clinics, acute care facilities, and nursing homes. They have been prominent centers for medical education and research in the United States. VA health care facilities—some in every state—account for nearly a million discharges from acute care and more than twenty-four million outpatient visits each year. A complex federal system of such size can be expected to have bureaucratic difficulties, and we do. The major question in 1990 centered on how to go about making this system work better for all its customers: the veterans we treat, the Congress, and the American taxpayers we serve.

Peter Drucker (1974) underscored the importance of this inquiry when he noted that American business often places too much emphasis on getting the right answer—the real issue should be asking the right question. Searching for the right answer to the wrong question is sometimes not very challenging, and finding it does not always improve our knowledge or our ability to make changes. In 1990, at the beginning of a reorganization prompted by James W. Holsinger Jr., M.D., the newly appointed chief medical director of the Veterans Health Administration (VHA), there was a general consensus about certain "right" answers but not much thought about whether we knew the proper questions. We were engaged in telling each other right answers to a limited range of questions and spent little time asking other questions. Nonetheless, one question seemed clear and right, and it was present in nearly every meeting: "What can we do to fix these problems?" The answer to that question varied among the different senior executives, who had varied levels of experience and different management styles.

As we pondered the issue of repairing the system, other questions began to arise: "What are we here to do?" "What exactly is the part that's broken?" "Where do we want to be in five or ten years?" These and similar questions led to our understanding that there were many areas that needed fixing and that everyone would have to be involved, not just the senior executives. That realization fit well with the impetus already under way for instituting total quality improvement (TQI) at VHA. We realized that perhaps the answer to "What can we do to fix these problems?" was "Implement TQI throughout the system." Plans for that implementation were already germinating, and the recognition by senior management of the magnitude of the problem added fuel and urgency to the process. For the plan to fit the circumstances, however, we needed to understand where we were as a system and how our national and local problems were generated and sustained. We needed a diagnosis before we could properly set out a course of treatment.

VHA's decision-making and resource management systems had been constructed over a half century before and had been rebuilt over the years by VHA headquarters and by local administrators with differing views of management and leadership. The challenges facing VHA's senior executives at the time of the 1990 reorganization included some very chronic conditions, dysfunctional behavior, and entrenched attitudes. These were what had evolved as "answers" to previous questions and circumstances. The history and structure of the organization had produced an aging bureaucracy with mild paranoia, sclerotic and arthritic limbs, a hidebound institutional memory, and an obvious decrease in vision and self-confidence. But the first wave of institutional testing ordered by top management in 1990 to diagnose the organization's ills uncovered a budding desire to improve both people's perception about its capabilities and the reality. Some VHA organs were clearly functioning very well—in fact they were true islands of excellence. And there were any number of others who wanted to be a part of change and improvement. Even though the prognosis seemed grim, the condition was certainly not terminal, and enthusiasm grew among the executives responsible for trying to devise a treatment plan for the organization.

Theory and practical experience, side by side, began to shape a plan that would address the organization's doldrums and apathy. The proposed plan of action would not be cheap, and it would not be a quick fix. The plan called for slow and steady doses of research, education, and encouragement, beginning with only a few parts of the organization. The therapy called for a rational increase in the dosing schedule and a broader spectrum of administration as the organization began to rally and show signs of improvement. A few years of treatment were anticipated before the patient would regain its strength and stature.

With all good intentions, the therapy was begun. Almost immediately it ran into problems, barriers, and delays. No one person was at fault, but still the delays mounted; the schedule slipped, and the few areas receiving treatment began to show some adverse reactions in addition to benefits. As the forward progress began to slow for the organization as a whole, there were a few organs that demanded more time and attention because of their own needs and success. Too much was at stake for the treatment team to become discouraged; each small victory gave them more heart. They found ways to get around the barriers and discovered means to effectively deliver higher treatment doses at a faster rate. The patient began to show systemic signs of improvement—sometimes so obvious that it was recognized by outsiders.

Even though the treatment course was successfully completed and the patient not only survived but clearly was the better for it, retrospective analysis showed how the plan could have been better, how some therapies worked better than others, and how the patient just needed more time to deal with the side effects of treatment before significant additional progress could be made. Thus some important lessons were learned about the course of treatment, and there were more lessons to come. Changes had to be made before the second, larger course was delivered.

Although the medical analogy in the previous paragraphs

seems to fit the situation reasonably well, the course of action VHA undertook when it inserted TQI across the system was not based on a medical construct. Rather, the plan, the consultant, and the basic approach were based on the industrial model of TQI, exemplified in the writings of Deming (Gitlow & Gitlow, 1987), Batalden (Batalden & Buchanan, 1989), and Berwick (1989). A key thrust in this model is the development of a culture that does not use data for punitive reasons but rather for detecting needed improvements and documenting them when they occur.

Berwick, Godfrey, and Roessner (1990) demonstrated the general applicability of the industrial model of TQI to the health care setting in their seminal work *Curing Health Care*. Nonetheless, there is another model of quality improvement, one more medically structured and familiar to health care professionals, that VHA might have chosen instead. The method of formulating scientific hypotheses, performing distribution analyses, and questioning and testing everything in the pursuit of ever-better medicine—what physicians and nurses are trained to do—has been identified as a "new" approach to quality in health care, called "the epidemiology of medical care" (Bowen, 1987). Donabedian (1990) agrees with this determination, saying, "A marriage between epidemiology and health care administration would be the emergence of a new health professional: one who might be called a clinical-performance epidemiologist."

What might have been different if VHA had taken the "medical," epidemiological route instead of the industrial one? Probably not very much at all—although the two camps suggest there are significant differences in their approach, they are actually quite similar. If there is a difference between the two methods, it probably lies in how they address the major interested consumer as the "patient" in the one and the "customer" in the other. Physicians are uncomfortable calling their patients "customers" and likely would have reacted less harshly to the epidemiologic terminology, but there are many other significant players on the health care team who do not have what could be described as a doctor-patient relationship with the people they serve. In the end, the strength of the effort's purpose—to make data-driven decisions, to focus on the real root of problems (processes, not people), and to allow and encourage all employees to join in improving the organization—

obviated the need to emphasize any particular method. In fact, much of what VHA decided in terms of the direction it would take on this journey was based upon the principle that TQI is simply good management; it is not a religion, and there is no Holy Writ, mantras, catechism, or sacred terminology—or priesthood.

Nevertheless, the importance of involving physicians in the TQI process from the very beginning has been stressed in the literature (Berwick, Godfrey, & Roessner, 1990), and we believed this was true. The original plan for the first phases of TQI implementation included thoroughly considered ways of addressing the physician audience at each individual hospital. We provided training for the physician consultants and gave them materials about the common questions physicians ask (with reasonable answers) and some examples of success stories from the medical field, including many from VHA experience. Nonetheless, we faced a difficult task early on. Physicians were reluctant even to attend TQI sessions focusing on the potential for improving care in their facility (self-regulated beepers are a salvation to the busy clinician). The questions and comments from those who did attend were familiar and common: "How will putting a team together help anything? I know what's wrong around here." "My patients are just older and sicker than anybody else's." "I don't have time to sit around talking about everybody else's job. If they would just do their job, we wouldn't have these problems."

A key part of our plan to create physician enthusiasm was to agree with them on one very key point, a point that is difficult for the industrial model to accept—health care ain't Honda. The industrial supplier can be required to provide raw materials in the purest form, milled to extreme tolerance and with virtually no variation; the substrate of health care walks in the door with the entire human range of variation. The concept of risk adjustment (taking the disease burden into account) makes an allowance for this difference, but this is not a concept taught in the original industrial TQI model. Once physicians feel that this obvious difference between the TQI model and their real-life experience is recognized and taken into account, their largest criticism of TQI concepts and the approach of making data-driven decisions is set aside.

Another important difference between the industrial and health care models of continuous improvement occurs at the "customer" interface. For most products, the interaction between the customer and the industry is through a trained salesman who is aware of the strengths of the product and is willing to not make a sale if the circumstances are disadvantageous. In health care, patients directly contact a wide variety of individuals, some highly trained and some not. The team effort in health care is out front and very visible to all. Further, the product of health care is quite personal; this is not an encounter either side can walk away from because the price is too high or the color scheme isn't right. Again, though, when physicians became aware that these differences were perceived by the quality improvement team, they became less defensive and were more readily drawn into the process.

Many individuals, inside and outside of health care, believe that physicians are too set in their ways to make changes; they think that the biggest challenge in bringing TQI into the health care arena will be to get physicians to change their behavior. In fact, it is remarkably easy to persuade physicians to change their mind. The education of physicians is based upon the scientific method. They are driven from day one to learn the reasons for disease—they seek the data behind the pathophysiology. Physicians, as a group, readily and often change their ways of approaching certain clinical circumstances. They read of a new technique, a new therapy, or a new approach to a thorny clinical problem, and they are generally willing to try it *if their present way of handling that circumstance is not satisfactory*. They may be unhappy with the current method for any number of reasons: it takes too long, their patients don't like it, or the outcomes are not what they would like. In these circumstances, physicians readily and quickly try a new approach. The same is true with TQI—when physicians are presented with key issues: the outcomes of the present situation are not acceptable, there is data to suggest that a better solution exists (or an opportunity exists to obtain such data), and the rest of the health care team wants and needs their input. In these circumstances, virtually every physician is interested in doing whatever is necessary to make a change for the better. Barriers of time and lost income associated with process improvement may require some innovative solutions, but often, if the approach is right, the physician becomes a part of that solution as well.

Another successful approach to involving physicians is to emphasize that the TQI approach is not foreign to their background and training. The elements of the Shewhart cycle ("Plan, Do, Check, Act," or PDCA) are familiar to all physicians (although they are expressed using a different terminology); testing hypotheses, gathering and analyzing data, trying new concepts and evaluating their usefulness are all part of the armamentarium of the physician. It would be unusual for physicians to resist the invocations that their patients need better outcomes, that a method for developing an improved process is in need of their input and participation, and that the driving force for change will be their own scientifically valid data. As we observed throughout the introduction of TQI into VHA, physicians were not impossible to recruit into the action; they needed to have their motivating factors clarified, and they were then usually ready to participate. We thought that the involvement of physicians was so critical that we put extra time and effort into the plan to develop special approaches to reaching them right from the beginning.

In a similar fashion, we are certainly convinced that the process of continuous improvement will lag and falter in any site where there is either inconsistent support from leadership or clear indifference. VA hospitals that made the most progress and attracted the most employees were those where the leadership clearly supported TQI concepts. This is not a new lesson, but perhaps there is a message in the widely diverse styles the different successful leaders exhibited. A common mystique is that there are "TQI kinds of people"; when probed, this opinion holds that leaders who will do well in the TQI environment are gregarious, friendly, outgoing and people-oriented. The actual findings, however, indicate that such characteristics, while often found in successful leaders, are not as predictive of success in implementing TQI in a hospital as honesty and a belief in people's ability to make data-driven changes. There is no "style" to TQI; it is a way of living and managing information and leading people, and it comes in all shapes and sizes.

We also became aware of some of the costs of TQI to the hospital workforce. Often, in the past, a worker could rise occasionally to confront a challenging situation and even get a reputation for being a problem solver with only a few successes a year. The continuous improvement expectation, however, is ever present, more like "what have you done for me lately?" This can be wearying to employees, regardless of their station. We learned that the process can cause burnout if the system expects too much from workers, whether they are leading a group, facilitating, teaching, or just being a team member. Continuous stress from high and demanding expectations can lead to organizational burnout as well. Individuals and organizations—whole hospitals—must be paced to make improvements gradually and not pushed as if perfection must be attained before the next holiday.

Two support mechanisms have shown promise in preventing both individual and organizational burnout. The first, and most easily embraced, is to teach and model reliance on teams. Teams are the strength of the TQI process, mostly because the collective ideas of a group are more valuable and more likely to succeed than those of a single individual. In the same way, the collective strength of a team, formal or not, can provide support to each of its members. The staff members involved in the selection of team members should be sensitive to the individual needs of the employees they select and be ready to give them time away from the process—no matter how valuable their services might be—in order to reassure them that they are part of a larger team, the system as a whole, that will carry the responsibility for continuing the improvement.

A second way of helping to lessen the likelihood of burnout is through a reward and recognition system. Burnout and discouragement occur more quickly when there is failure or where there is no recognition of success. Others have taught the value of celebrating the failures in a change process; we also believe that those who do so will maintain the spirit of the workforce. Such celebration of failure carries many important messages: failure is not fatal, now that we have clearly identified a wrong way we won't waste any more time doing that, people are still more important than the process, and so on. Rewards for success should reinforce the concepts and precepts of the continuous improvement model as well. Specifically, the rewards should be given to the team and not to individuals (not even to the "MVP"). There is no more public way to endorse the usefulness and effectiveness of teamwork in a facility than to recognize the team for its success. At least once, we heard someone in an audience watching a team award ceremony ask, "How do I get on one of *those* teams?"

At the beginning of this chapter I used a medical analogy to describe the problem facing VHA and its response to that problem. Just as in a patient care process, the next step in VHA's TQI effort is to evaluate the outcome. Did the treatment work? Were there side effects? Should we try this again, or should we change the process?

A major difficulty in obtaining physician participation in TQI is providing some reasonable estimation that patient care will be improved as a result of the changes being contemplated. Just as those involved in the National Demonstration Project found, it is appealing and easy to focus on administrative issues rather than patient care outcomes. Such behavior is shortsighted and self-defeating. Even though we may legitimately argue that it is important to improve administrative processes, too often the reason we are improving them is because they are easier to address. There is often better data for administrative processes than for clinical processes. But focusing our attention there is very much like looking for our lost car keys under the streetlight. It's true, the light is better there, but the keys were lost back up the street, in the dark, and looking for them under the streetlight will never be successful. To enlist and maintain the interest and active participation of physicians and other clinicians, the improvement processes in a hospital must have direct patient applicability. Sometimes that applicability is not immediately evident, but the search for and identification of the clinical relevance of TQI activities is highly rewarding for everyone.

As an example, many VA hospitals identified chart retrieval as a problem in their outpatient clinics. Physicians often complained that the unavailability of a patient's medical record when they saw the patient compromised the quality of care. When the process of chart filing and retrieval was examined and improved, the measure of improvement reported by facilities was simply the difference between the retrieval rate before and after the intervention ("It was 67 percent but now it is 89 percent"). Such measures are relatively easy to obtain and bear some connection to the original complaint, but they are, at best, only indirect measures of the quality of patient care. The staff at some hospitals, when encouraged to do so, began to look beyond the retrieval rate to determine whether the presence of the medical record at the time of a patient examination was associated with significant improvements in the patient's outcomes. They examined measures such as the rate of laboratory testing, drug prescribing, or procedure performance to determine if the presence of information in the medical record was a factor in dissuading providers from performing additional diagnostic tests. They also tried to evaluate the impact that the presence of the chart might have on reducing drug interactions from new prescriptions; admissions for adverse drug reactions were part of the tracking data. Such information will ultimately be more convincing to physicians and others that TQI efforts are of value to the patients they treat and are not simply a way of improving administrative procedures in the hospital.

Another set of problems for the implementation of TQI within VHA related to the original construct for headquarters' role in the program. This role contributed to the difficulties in obtaining a clinical focus. The artificial distinction between the administrative focus of the Office of Resource Management and the clinical focus of the Office of Quality Management in developing and overseeing a pilot TQI program created confusion in the field. Many facilities, following a long tradition, tried to mirror the central administrative structure in their hospital (an action that was endorsed or in some instances suggested by the paid consultants). In these hospitals, the existing quality management activities became isolated from the TQI activities, with the result that improvement activities became increasingly nonclinical. This complicated the recruitment of physicians into total quality improvement and increased the need for explicit efforts to get and maintain their input and active participation. While these actions were successful to a degree, the duplicate administrative structures and parallel activities, at times, deflected some of the energy and enthusiasm of employees. Often the introduction of total quality improvement ("three-letter Q") methods into the hospital conflicted with the beliefs of clinicians and administrators who thought they were already deeply involved in "quality" in the form of quality assurance ("two-letter Q"). Some consultants made this situation worse by trying to compare two-letter Q (a program for gathering and measuring data) to three-letter Q (a philosophy of managing data), thereby creating further uncertainty, especially in the eyes of the very clinicians that were needed to make TQI activities relevant.

In this regard, then, there should be no artificial separation of these two activities, especially not in the organization chart. Health care organizations that assign separate boxes (on an organization chart) to the two-letter Q and three-letter Q functions will have significant difficulty keeping any clinical significance in the TQI part of the activity. If these two functions are organized as competing activities, a great deal of time and energy will be wasted throughout the organization. VHA learned that lesson during the initial phase of its TQI implementation and made substantive structural, cultural, and organizational changes to address the problem in subsequent phases.

Thirty-eight hospitals participated in VHA's TQI implementation, and their experiences, now exceeding thirty-six months per hospital, are reviewed and reported in this book. Many teams have been chartered and empowered; scores of processes have been charted and reengineered, and the movement has spread throughout the entire VHA system of 172 hospitals and all its clinics. Two electronic databases have been created to track progress—one deals with the topics addressed by individual process improvement teams and the structure of those teams, and the other tracks a variety of improvements made by the teams.

As VHA begins to solidify its gains following its national rollout of TQI, the lingering and recurrent question is "So what?" We believe this may be the right question for the future. Most important, we think, is the effect TQI will have on the care we provide our veteran patients. Are they better off now than they were before we began the TQI implementation? Is there reason to believe that the progress we have made so far will continue to improve their care, their satisfaction, and their outcomes?

But just like a child, who must learn to walk before learning to run, the VHA health care system had to learn to "walk the TQI walk and talk the TQI talk." This book is about learning to walk and learning to talk. As a system, VHA has not yet learned how to walk, although some individual hospitals are already beginning to run.

Some may wonder why we have written a book on learning how to walk, when running is so much more exciting. As any parent knows, learning to walk involves trial and error and bumps and maybe a few bruises and scrapes. VHA's TQI journey has certainly had its share of bumps, bruises, and scrapes. Reading about these may not allow others to completely avoid them, but it can at least demonstrate that bumps and bruises are normal concomitants of any TQI journey. The foremost lesson of VHA's TQI effort is that TQI is not easy and will not occur without some pain. Knowing just that much beforehand may make the pain seem more normal and possibly help those who are easily discouraged to keep the faith and persevere.

This book, then, is not a how-to book on TQI, nor is it an evaluation of how well (or poorly) we implemented it. Rather, it presents, in a somewhat anecdotal manner, lessons learned in the process of implementing TQI in a large, government-run health care organization. As one might expect, what happened was not necessarily what the framers, planners, and practitioners expected or desired. But it shows what *can* happen in TQI, and in that context lie valuable lessons, not only for future generations in VHA but also for health care practitioners in general. It is left to them to apply the "So what?" question to the continuing quest for excellence in health care.

References

Batalden, P. B., & Buchanan, E. D. (1989). Industrial models of quality improvement. In N. Goldfield & D. B. Nash (Eds.), *Providing health care: The challenge to clinicians* (pp. 133–159). Philadelphia: American College of Physicians.

Berwick, D. M. (1989). Continuous improvement as an ideal in health care. *New England Journal of Medicine, 320,* 53–56.

Berwick, D. M., Godfrey, A. B., & Roessner, J. (1990). *Curing health care: New strategies for quality improvement.* San Francisco: Jossey-Bass.

Bowen, O. R. (1987). Shattuck lecture: What is quality care? *New England Journal of Medicine, 316,* 1578–1579.

Donabedian, A. (1990). Contributions of epidemiology to quality assessment and monitoring. *Infection Control and Hospital Epidemiology, 11,* 117–121.

Drucker, P. F. (1974). *Managing in turbulent times.* New York: Harper & Row.

Gitlow, H. S., & Gitlow, S. J. (1987). *The Deming guide to quality and competitive position.* Englewood Cliffs, NJ: Prentice-Hall.

Chapter Two

Assessing Our History and Traditions

Galen L. Barbour

The bureaucracy that confronted proponents of total quality improvement (TQI) at the Veterans Health Administration (VHA) in the early 1990s was formidable—almost intimidating. The status quo was preferred to anything but small, incremental change. "This too will pass" was an almost reflexive response to change by bureaucrats conditioned to bend with the political and organizational winds but never break. VHA's culture had evolved over the years to successfully adapt to the forces surrounding it. But in government, adaptation often includes compromise, and the compromises made over the years at VHA produced a health care system best described as hidebound. Anachronisms were endemic. VHA facilities and programs were located in places that defied logic in the 1990s, and attempts to realign the system and make it more rational were invariably ground down to cosmetic proportions.

Culture and traditions are a source of both strength and weakness in an organization. On the one hand, they give the members of an organization a sense of pride, purpose, and stability. On the other hand, they can stifle needed change. New employees (perhaps with fresh ideas) in VHA quickly learn that change is viewed with caution, and anecdotes abound to convince the neophyte that most ideas for change come and go without making a substantive impact.

The longer an organization exists, the greater the power of its traditions; this power can work to either the benefit or the detriment of an organization. It benefits the organization by providing stability and staying power. It hurts it if that stability forestalls change that is needed to flourish (or even to survive). For these reasons, it is instructive to digress briefly in this chapter and describe where the VHA health care system came from, what it looks like, and what it has accomplished. With this knowledge, one can better understand the challenge that has faced the early proponents of TQI in VHA.

The tradition of caring for veterans has deep roots in the American psyche. Almost a century and a half before the formation of the United States, the American colonies established statutory benefits for veterans injured in military actions (Gronvall, 1989). From this beginning arose America's proud tradition of honoring and caring for those who have worn its uniform. Plymouth Colony, following the English tradition of providing monetary benefits for those injured in the service of the Crown, passed a law in 1636 establishing such benefits in the colony; later this law was adopted by the new nation, which assigned the federal government responsibility for the veterans of the Revolutionary War. In 1811 Congress authorized the construction of the U.S. Naval Asylum in Philadelphia, established to provide government-funded institutional care for veterans. In 1833 the asylum became the first "pre-paid closed panel group health plan" in America (Gronvall, 1989). The U.S. Soldiers' and Airmen's Home in Washington, D.C., was created by Congress in 1851 to serve veterans of the U.S. Army. It provided domiciliary care primarily, but general medical and hospital care were also provided. After the Civil War, the National Home for Disabled Volunteer Soldiers was created by Congress to deal with veterans' health care needs. This represented the first large-scale effort to care for U.S. veterans. Like the Soldiers' and Airmen's Home, the National Home system was primarily domiciliary in nature but also provided medical care to ambulatory patients and arranged for hospital care for those in need. In 1919 Congress created a federally funded system of veterans' hospitals, to be operated by the Public Health Service, explicitly to deal with the influx of veterans returning after the Great War. Federal funding allowed for the purchase of some existing hospitals and the construction of others to meet the expected need. By 1920, the Public Health Service had opened forty-six new hospi-

tals, with the capacity to care for eighty-seven thousand hospital-
ized veterans (Adkins, 1967).

The idea of providing veterans with health benefits actually
arose from the issue of worker's compensation, which was viewed
as especially important for workers injured in the industrial effort
to support the war. Business leaders around the country recognized
the need and propriety of providing health insurance to workers,
just as they had provided them with life insurance and pensions. It
was "just plain horse-sense" (Stevens, 1991). As a result of con-
scription in World War I, the U.S. government had become a major
employer. And its workers—its soldiers and sailors—were involved
in an especially unhealthy and dangerous occupation. As a consequence of these forces, veterans of the U.S. military were provided
health benefits by the War Risk Insurance Act of 1914 (which was
primarily aimed at providing disability benefits). These actions
came on the heels of a rising recognition of the federal government's responsibility for the health and welfare of military con-
scripts and an acknowledgement that such responsibility does not
cease at the end of hostile action. In 1921, aware of the rapidly increasing need for veterans' care and the disparity between its efforts in this area and other functions of the Public Health Service,
Congress created the independent Veterans Bureau to oversee the
military hospital system.

The system grew slowly. The Veterans Administration (VA) was
created in 1930 by combining three other federal agencies that
provided services to veterans: the National Home for Disabled Volunteer Soldiers, the Veterans Bureau, and the Bureau of Pensions.
At that time there were forty-seven hospitals in the system, with an
aggregate capacity of 22,700 beds. Over the next fifteen years,
America provided its veterans with more and more services
through a growing bureaucracy, composed largely of former members of the military. At the close of the World War II, the enormous
task of readying the system to handle the influx of veterans returning from Europe and Asia required some major changes in the
system itself.

Veterans of that era and succeeding eras owe a huge debt of
gratitude to two men who, in today's TQI parlance, "reengineered"
the VA health care system. First, the team of Omar Bradley and
Paul Magnuson, M.D., proposed a substantive change to the Civil

Service Act—to create a separate personnel system for hiring physicians, to get around the red tape of the federal bureaucracy. Second, they shepherded a partnership between America's medical schools (who had a difficult problem—doctors without patients) and the VA (who had patients without doctors). These changes brought great benefits to veterans and to American medicine (Magnuson, 1960). Adopting the academic approach to the practice of medicine in the VA led to the development of research programs that have contributed much to medical science.

The Veterans Administration was composed of three divisions: the Department of Medicine and Surgery (DM&S), which delivered health care; the Department of Veterans Benefits (DVB), which administered benefits; and the Department of Memorial Affairs (DMA), which oversaw burials and cemeteries. In 1989 the VA was elevated by Congress to cabinet level and thus renamed the Department of Veterans Affairs, known simply as "VA" (without "the"). Like the old Veterans Administration, VA had three divisions, providing the same services as before but called by different names: DM&S became the Veterans Health Services and Research Administration (VHS&RA), DVB became the Veterans Benefits Administration (VBA), and DMA became the National Cemetery System (NCS). In 1991 Congress renamed VHS&RA the Veterans Health Administration, or VHA.

Just as yesterday's medical breakthroughs become today's routine medical procedures, so have yesterday's institutional stars become today's workaday hospitals. Today's VA hospitals are not widely regarded as research institutions, in spite of the fact that VHA researchers have contributed with distinction to the field of medicine. Although two VHA researchers have been awarded the Nobel Prize for medicine, the general public remains unaware of the medical discoveries and advances produced by VHA-funded research over the years. The two Nobel laureates, Dr. Rosalyn Yalow (Bronx VA medical center), recognized for her pioneering work with radioimmunoassays (Yalow & Berson, 1973, 1971), and Dr. Andrew Schally (New Orleans VA medical center), recognized for his research on brain hormones (Schally, Bowers, Redding, & Barrett, 1966; Schally, Nair, Redding, & Arimura, 1971), opened the doors for enormous advances in their fields through their VHA-related endeavors. Other significant medical advances and innovations produced by VHA researchers include the CAT scanner (Oldendorf, 1961); the cardiac pacemaker (Chardack, Gage, & Greatbatch, 1960); and successful methods for treating hypertension (Materson and others, 1993), tuberculosis (Tucker, 1960), and schizophrenia (Casey and others, 1961). VHA researchers were also responsible for collecting the data that led to the recognition of the role of surgery in treating coronary artery disease (Peduzzi & Hultgren, 1979; Lewis and others, 1983) and for a host of prosthetic devices and techniques for use by amputees and stroke victims. The parade continues—VHA contributions in the past few years include proof of the effectiveness of laser surgery in treating prostate cancer (Kabalin & Gill, 1993), new protocols for the timing of drug therapy in treating AIDS (Hamilton and others, 1992), demonstrations of the benefits of adult day care centers in caring for the aged (Hendrick & Branch, 1993), and new directions for the future of geriatric assessment (Deyo, Applegate, Kramer, & Meehan, 1991). VHA has just been granted a patent application number for a mobile laboratory cart that performs most common laboratory tests at the point of care. This invention will help hospitals save on personnel and resource costs and reduce duplicate testing. As with the discoveries made by VHA investigators in past decades, these recent contributions are likely to benefit all patients and practitioners, not just veterans and VHA doctors.

In addition, the affiliation between VHA and U.S. medical schools has had a positive impact on American medical education. VHA academic affiliates have fulfilled their promise for recruiting and retaining highly qualified professionals as well as for creating an environment of academic inquiry that builds expectations of constant improvement and high-quality outcomes. Recognizing the value of such liaisons, Congress legislated the Manpower Grant program in the 1970s, creating five new medical schools in the United States with five VA medical centers as the parent teaching institution. Currently, 130 VHA facilities are affiliated with 105 of the nation's 126 medical schools and all 55 of its dental schools. More than thirty thousand medical residents and twenty-two thousand medical students train in VHA facilities every year in traditional mainstream programs.

In addition, VHA's academic support for specialty training programs in nonaccredited fields has developed a cadre of specialists committed to academic excellence. In the area of geriatrics, VHA's contributions have been critical to geriatric medicine's being recognized as a specialty by the Accreditation Council for Graduate Medical Education (ACGME) in 1988 and geriatric psychiatry's reaching ACGME-accreditation status in 1994. VHA has since supported other needed nonaccredited training programs, providing clinical training and research in the care and rehabilitation of spinal cord–injured patients and in the field of substance abuse, psychiatric research into the biologic bases of mental illnesses, and a cooperative venture with the Robert Wood Johnson Foundation to fund clinical scholars in the study of health services and health care policy. Other areas in which VHA is providing support for academic training include ambulatory care, clinical pharmacology, schizophrenia research, dental research, traumatic brain injury research, women's health issues, and medical informatics. Each of these programs will train future researchers and caregivers for all Americans, not just veterans.

However, the VHA bureaucracy did not always keep pace with other changes in health care delivery. It was not until 1970 that VA regulations allowed for the care of ambulatory patients other than to obviate the need for hospitalization or for post-discharge care. By 1990 the momentum toward ambulatory care had gained new life in the nonfederal sector as a means of delivering more cost-efficient care, but VHA, following long-established traditions, was still planning to build hospitals and operating rooms, not clinics and ambulatory surgery suites. Part of this resulted from the continued desire of individual members of Congress to place VA hospitals in their districts (Stevens, 1991, p. 297), and part of it was the result of the tedious and slow process of contracting for and building a major new hospital.

Even so, since the late 1970s the total number of VA facilities has remained nearly constant; the changes in the system have come from changes in the expectations of its customers—both patients and Congress—and changes in the practice of American medicine. In 1995 there were 172 medical centers, or hospitals, in the VHA system. Eighteen of those centers, however, were consolidated under a single administrative structure, creating ten dual-division hospitals. These consolidations, made for streamlining and personnel-reduction purposes, reduced the number of distinct facilities to 162 by the end of 1995. However they are organized, VHA facilities account for nine hundred thousand to one million acute care discharges each year. There are 310 outpatient clinics in the VHA system, and they handle twenty-four to twenty-five million visits each year. There are also twenty-seven domiciliaries (direct descendants of the National Homes), which each year provide care, vocational training, and rehabilitation for homeless or needy veterans, in addition, veterans receive long-term care in some of the nation's finest nursing homes.

The Department of Veterans Affairs employs 240,000 people, from the groundskeepers, benefits clerks, and maintenance workers who keep the physical plants and cemeteries functioning to the hospital directors, physicians, and nurses who maintain the delivery and care systems. Approximately one in every thousand Americans works for VA. About 12 percent of all U.S. medical residency positions in internal medicine, surgery, and psychiatry are directly funded by VHA, and those physicians-in-training work each day in VHA facilities across the nation. Well over 50 percent of the actively practicing physicians in the United States received some portion of their training in a VHA facility, where they contributed to the quality care that is regularly delivered there.

Although the number of veterans is steadily declining in the United States, the number that seek care from VHA remains relatively constant, approximately 10 per cent of the total veteran population in 1994. That group is largely composed of individuals with no health insurance and low incomes (less than $15,000 per year, $18,000 if married). VHA's role in caring for these individuals is to provide a safety net, removing a significant burden of otherwise uncompensated care from the medical community and society. This need is likely to increase in the future, in spite of the fact that veterans, as a class of citizens, have attained a higher level of education, higher income, and lower unemployment rate than the national average.

VHA employees often refer to the fact that VHA is the largest health care system in the world, based on number of facilities and beds. In fact, VHA resembles a "system" of health care in the same way that the former Yugoslavia resembles a country—both consist of balkanized functions and geographic sites that war continually with one another over resources. The bureaucracy of VHA was structured along military lines of "command and control." Similar to the "silo" effects seen in nonfederal agencies, the internally focused divisions, or "services," in every VHA facility seem constantly to be fighting a battle for resources. Not only does VHA and each of its components work from a fixed budget, but financial constraints also mean straight-line budgeting—no new programs can be created (nor, for that matter, can existing ones be significantly altered) without taking resources from somewhere else in the system. Each service and each facility feels the current belt-tightening in Washington; they respond by planning how to continue their current services, not by planning expansions or investigating where to take risks in developing new programs or activities.

As VHA has begun pushing its cost-reduction campaign systemwide, it has become apparent that its effects are not salutary. An initial attempt to bring rational thought to the budgeting process involved using the Resource Allocation Model (RAM), which is based in large part on the diagnosis-related groupings (DRG) and weighted–work unit theory. But calculations based on work load reporting under this system had several unintended effects. First, because of errors and omissions in the work load reports from the first year, redistribution of funds caused some major shifts in supportable employment. The use of two-year-old data in calculating future budgets also meant that inflation was not properly accounted for. Thus future budgets were eroded before they even began, often leading to two categories of VA hospitals under the new system: losers (those who lost money) and nonwinners (those who did not get any additional money). Further, as should have been expected, a work load–based reimbursement system quickly led to increased admissions, outpatient visits, tests, and procedures. This not only devalued the weighted–work unit approach but also moved practitioners and the entire system away from cost-efficiency.

A major additional effect of VHA's cost-containment efforts was a reduction in the time patients were allowed to stay in the hospital. As the average length of stay fell across the system, more and more beds went unoccupied. In any form of managed care, an empty bed is a good bed; thus this was seen as a laudable goal. Critics of VHA, however, began to point to the empty beds as evidence that there was less and less need for the entire system; the corresponding increase in the outpatient work load was often ignored, as if VHA were providing only inpatient care. A confounding issue at this time was VHA's practice of charging a different "service" with the care of inpatients from the "service" that cared for outpatients, even though both were cared for under the same roof. As a result of the bureaucracy's lack of focus on the result of care and its overattention to the process of care and where it occurs, VHA facilities had no incentive to shift their money and manpower from inpatient care areas to outpatient care areas to match the changes in work load.

Internally, VHA employees believe that they and their fellow workers are hardworking professionals (just like in other hospitals). They often share anecdotes about great "saves" with one another and then generalize those experiences to their particular institution. At other times they gripe and grumble about other service's employees not making their own job easier. Rarely do employees share laudatory anecdotes about the VHA system as a whole. Patients often encounter both good and bad experiences, however, and alternately praise and criticize their care and experience in the system.

Externally, there are different beliefs about the quality of care in VHA—including views that are different from those held within VHA and different from those held by Congress just a few decades ago. Media attention, focused on episodes of bad outcomes from VHA care—often single cases or a few similar cases from one facility—has carried with it the suggestion that all VHA care is substandard. In a similar vein, members of Congress have used committee hearings to air isolated stories of bad VHA care (often true, regrettably) as they "champion" veterans' rights to high-quality care (by criticizing the professionals and administrators of the system charged with delivering that care). This picture of VHA care, presented by the investigative media or the investigative arm of Congress (whose "duty" is to find fault and error), suggests that all care delivered by VHA is below the standard found in the private sector. This "knothole" view of the issue often ignores the fact that the VHA care being criticized is no different from that provided, often by the same physicians, at the highly regarded affiliated university hospital next door. The overall effect of this criticism, however, has been to make the employees of VHA feel that their individual contributions are neither noticed nor valued; they feel that they are painted with the same brush used to criticize VHA generally on the basis of a few instances of poor care or bad outcomes. Understandably, morale is often low.

When Jim Holsinger became chief medical director in 1990, what seemed to be most needed was a reliable way to measure the quality of various aspects of the system and a workable plan to use those measurements to produce improvements across the system. In terms of measurement, what was needed was both a standard and a comparative. A fairly well-held belief at the time was that "quality is in the eyes of the beholder." By this most meant that quality means so many different things to different people that no one could possibly establish measures that would satisfy everyone. Interestingly enough, it was not common among those who discussed this issue to think of patients as "beholders."

The development of any system of measurement depends on a clear definition of what is to be measured. VHA wrestled with this concept and finally produced a working definition of health care quality to be used for measurement and improvement. That definition says that quality health care is care that is *needed* and delivered in a manner that is *competent, caring, cost-efficient* and *timely* and that *minimizes risk* and *achieves achievable benefits*. These seven attributes were further defined and used to evaluate the measures of quality then in use. Broadly speaking, VHA measures in 1990 focused on acute inpatient care, almost entirely medical or surgical. There was little to no measurement of outpatient care or psychiatric care, nor was there any good measure of patients' opinions of care. Furthermore, virtually all of the measurement capability for quality-of-care issues developed since then have been based on this needs assessment.

Equally important to the development of believable measures of quality was the development of a capability for process improvement, both locally and nationally. The balkanization of the system, including the "fee-basis" reimbursement scheme, made the improvement of cross-hospital processes very difficult. There also was no accepted, endorsed strategy or lexicon for addressing a national issue such as process improvement. National educational programs were slow to develop, very costly, and not necessarily germane to the issue; there was not a good, reliable method to roll out systemwide change. Further, the large, bureaucratic, military-like structure of the organization, which was the target of constant public criticism, had not involved its employees in problem solving and thus could not now turn to them for assistance. Nonetheless, there was not a major disaster or a looming catastrophe that pushed VHA into adopting TQI principles. The leadership style of the new chief medical director, James W. Holsinger Jr., M.D., and the positive experiences of John Fears, director at the Hines VA hospital in Chicago, melded with the changes occurring in the rest of the profession and emphasized the need to find a more effective strategy. Recognizing that this need called for an amazing transformation to fit in with the mainstream of health care in the United States, VHA undertook to bring an entirely new way of thinking to its individual hospitals and to the system: processes are the problem, not people. People are the answer, not the cause, of our problems; teams of people are better able to solve problems; decisions are better when based in fact than in guesswork or opinion; and all our processes can be improved. VHA leadership was ready to accept the formidable challenge of changing the way this leviathan did business: we were going to become immersed and involved in TQI.

References

Adkins, R. E. (1967). *Medical care of veterans.* Washington, DC: U.S. Government Printing Office.

Casey, J. F., Bennett, I. F., Lindley, C. J., Hollister, L., Gordon, M. H., & Springer, N. N. (1961). Drug therapy in schizophrenia: A controlled study of the relative effectiveness of chlorpromazine, promazine, phenobarbital, and placebo. *Archives of General Psychiatry, 4,* 381–389.

Chardack, W. M., Gage, A. A., & Greatbatch, W. (1960). A transistorized self-oriented implantable pacemaker for the long-term correction of complete heart block. *Surgery, 48,* 643–654.

Deyo, R., Applegate, W. B., Kramer, A., & Meehan, S. (1991). The future of geriatric assessment. (Pt. 2). [Special issue]. *Journal of the American Geriatric Society, 39*(Suppl.).

Gronvall, J. A. (1989). The VA's affiliation with academic medicine: An emergency post-war strategy becomes a permanent partnership. *Academic Medicine, 64,* 61–66.

Hamilton, J. D., Hartigan, P. M., Simberkoff, M. S., Day, P. L., Diamond, G. R., Dickinson, G. M., Drusano, G. L., Egorin, M. J., George, W. L.,

Gordin, F. M., & Associates. (1992). A controlled trial of early versus late treatment with zidovudine in symptomatic human immunodeficiency virus infection. *New England Journal of Medicine, 326*, 437–443.

Hendrick, S. C., & Branch, L. G. (Eds.). (1993). Adult day care evaluation study [Special issue]. *Medical Care, 31*(Suppl.), 9.

Kabalin, J. N., & Gill, H. S. (1993). Urolase laser prostatectomy in patients on warfarin anticoagulation: A safe treatment alternative for bladder outlet obstruction. *Urology, 42*, 738–740.

Lewis, H. D., Jr., Davis, J. W., Archibald, D. G., Steinke, W. E., Smitherman, T. C., Doherty, J. E. III, Schnaper, H. W., LeWinter, M. M., Linares, E., Pouget, J. M., Sabharwal, S. C., Chesler, E., & DeMots, H. (1983). Protective effects of aspirin against acute myocardial infarction and death in men with unstable angina. *New England Journal of Medicine, 309*, 396–403.

Magnuson, P. B. (1960). *Ring the night bell.* Boston: Little, Brown.

Materson, B. J., Reda, D. J., Cushman, W. C., Massie, B. M., Freis, E. D., Kochar, M. S., Hamburger, R. J., Fye, C., Lakshman, R., Gottdiener, J., & Associates. (1993). Single-drug therapy for hypertension in men: A comparison of six antihypertensive agents with placebo. *New England Journal of Medicine, 328*(13), 959–961.

Oldendorf, W. H. (1961). Isolated flying-spot detection of radiodensity discontinuities: displaying the internal structural pattern of a complex object. *IRE Transactions on Bio-medical Electronics, 8*, 68–72.

Peduzzi, P., & Hultgren, H. (1979). Effect of medical vs. surgical treatment on symptoms in stable angina pectoris: The Veterans Administration cooperative study of surgery for coronary arterial occlusive disease. *Circulation, 60*, 888–900.

Schally, A. V., Bowers, C. Y., Redding T. W., & Barrett, J. F. (1966). Isolation of thyrotropin releasing factor (TRF) from porcine hypothalamus. *Biochemical and Biophysical Research Communications, 25*, 165–169.

Schally, A. V., Nair, R. M., Redding, T. W., & Arimura, A. (1971). Isolation of the LH and FSH-releasing hormone from porcine hypothalami. *Journal of Biological Chemistry, 246*, 7230–7236.

Stevens, R. (1991). Can the government govern? Lessons from the formation of the Veterans Administration. *Journal of Health Politics, Policy and Law, 16*, 281–305.

Tucker, W. B. (1960). The evolution of the cooperative studies in the chemotherapy of tuberculosis of the Veterans Administration and armed forces of the USA. *Advanced Tuberculosis Research, 10*, 1–68.

Yalow, R. S., & Berson, S. A. (1971). Size heterogeneity of immunoreactive human ACTH in plasma and in extracts of pituitary glands and ACTH-producing thymoma. *Biochemical Biophysical Research Communications, 44,* 439–445.

Yalow, R. S., & Berson, S. A. (1973). Characteristics of "Big ACTH" in human plasma and pituitary extracts. *Journal of Clinical Endocrinology and Metabolism, 36,* 415–423.

Chapter Three

Borrowing from Industry: Bringing Total Quality Improvement to Health Care

Richard R. Lussier

In the last decade of the twentieth century, the monolithic Veterans Health Administration (VHA) finds itself facing more tough challenges than ever before. Fundamental changes are taking place in health care, changes that are increasingly difficult to ignore. No longer is there comfort in the phrase "this too shall pass"—the forces driving change are now too strong and too persistent. Huge, complicated questions are demanding answers from VHA managers. How will VHA survive the economic restructuring of the American health care system? Will it be able to make the transition from a hospital-based inpatient care system to an ambulatory care system, where capital assets (like hospitals) are considered a liability? How will research and medical education survive when they are seen only as cost centers? How will the medical profession in general meet the demand for primary care practitioners and still incorporate specialists and subspecialists into the spectrum of care? How will it include patients and their family members in the health care delivery system? How will physicians effectively recognize and meet their customers' needs? How will the marketing of health care products and services be handled in the new environment? And perhaps most critical of all, how will the quality of clinical care be maintained while all these other changes are taking place? Each of these challenges is a thread in the banner of health care reform. Clearly, Walton must have had times like this in mind when she said, "The status quo will not do" (Walton, 1986, p. 57).

Because VHA faces the same challenges facing all of American health care, it will have to change along with it. The political, cultural, and economic environment surrounding VHA will demand change. The hospitals and health care systems that survive will be the ones that are able to meet the challenges listed above—and do so with cost-effective answers. Containing the spiraling costs of health care is an obvious driving need behind the call for major change in the American health care system; but there is also a push for accountability on the part of the profession, and that will require meeting the challenges in a manner that maintains or improves the current high state of quality in health care delivery (Relman, 1988). This demand for accountability calls for still another transition, from the practice of attempting to ensure quality by retrospective data analysis to developing processes designed to steadily improve care outcomes. The new impetus to develop measures that drive continuous improvement in health care is only the most recent in a long and historic series of efforts by society and the medical profession to improve the quality of medical care. One of the mechanisms selected to ensure accountability in VHA has existed in the private sector for years: total quality management (TQM), whose principles evolved out of industry's attempts to create the best products at the best prices.

The earliest quality assurance efforts were born in the workplace and probably took the form of inspections. From ancient times until the early 1900s, quality was "assured" by inspecting products after they were created; the inspector or customer determined, often with only implicit criteria, whether the product met a certain standard or was fit for the purpose for which it was created. Obviously this methodology created some degree of waste, and sometimes it allowed serious imperfections to reach the final stage of production before detection—occasionally with disastrous results.

The first significant change in this process was introduced by Henry Ford and Frederick Taylor during the 1890s. Their fundamental change was to assign primary responsibility for inspection to an individual trained in explicit criteria for reviewing the work of others (Walton, 1986, p. 9). Although this move created a greater standardization in quality assurance methodologies and, by extension, a greater consistency in the final product, the process still consisted of inspecting products that were essentially complete. Faults could only be detected, not prevented.

In the mid-1920s the work of Walter Shewhart, a scientist at what would become Bell Laboratories, began to bring the entire inspection approach into question. In 1931, Shewhart wrote a seminal work, *The Economic Control of the Quality of Manufactured Product,* that suggested a revolutionary concept to manufacturers. He recommended that companies not spend time and effort detecting and repairing flaws in their final products but that they instead try to identify and fix flaws in the work processes that produced those products. His basic premise was that proper control of the process of production was more important than inspection in ensuring and improving quality. Shewhart's principles were applied by both British and American industry during World War II in the manufacture of matériel, and they proved substantially effective (Berwick, Godfrey, & Roessner, 1990, p. 31).

At the end of the war, Japanese industry was devastated. Products marked "Made in Japan" were uniformly inferior to those made in other industrialized nations; Japanese businesses were eager to make whatever changes were needed to become competitive in the world market. They turned to some of the American leaders of the productivity movement and asked for their help and assistance in reasserting Japan's market share. Dr. W. Edwards Deming, a student of Shewhart, further developed his teacher's technique, adding statistical evaluation of variations as a means of understanding root causes and pointing the way to necessary improvements. Deming and Joseph M. Juran applied these refined principles in postwar Japanese industries, substantially boosting the quality improvement effort there.

Based on this experience, Deming developed a list of fourteen key principles of his philosophy of quality improvement (see Exhibit 3.1). That list became a polestar to the recovering Japanese business and manufacturing communities, and it became nearly as famous in the United States as American industry began adapting the concepts to their processes and products.

Juran brought the discipline and rigor of his engineering and law background to the problem of how to revitalize Japanese

Exhibit 3.1. Deming's Fourteen Principles
of Quality Improvement.

1. Drive out fear.

2. Eliminate quotas and numerical goals.

3. Break down barriers between departments.

4. Eliminate inspections. Build things right the first time.

5. Institute a vigorous program of education and self-improvement.

6. Remove barriers that rob workers of pride in their workmanship.

7. Institute leadership to help people do a better job.

8. Eliminate slogans, exhortations, and production targets.

9. Adopt a new philosophy for change.

10. End the practice of awarding business on the basis of price alone. Choose a single supplier and build a long-term relationship with them on the basis of loyalty and trust.

11. Improve constantly and forever the system of production and service.

12. Put everybody to work to accomplish the transformation.

13. Institute job training.

14. Create constancy of purpose toward improving products and services, to become competitive, to stay in business, and to provide jobs.

Source: Adapted from Walton, 1986, pp. 34–36.

industry. Between the two of them, Deming and Juran were largely responsible for the incredible turnaround in the Japanese business world. They accomplished this basically by emphasizing the need to prevent errors during the production process rather than to inspect the quality of the finished product. During the 1950s, Japanese business leaders and workers incorporated the concepts of Deming and Juran into a concept called *kaizen,* the continuous search for opportunities to improve every process. Incredibly, in spite of the success he enjoyed in Japan, Deming remained virtually unknown in the United States.

In 1978, Detroit automobile executives searching for ways to stem the decline of their market share consulted with Deming. They learned of his remarkable accomplishments in helping

Japanese companies increase their productivity by focusing on the quality of the manufacturing process rather than that of the final product.

The late 1970s and early 1980s were marked by the publication of four key resources that sparked the TQM revolution. *Juran's Quality Control Handbook* and Philip Crosby's *Quality Is Free* were first published in 1979; they were soon followed by Deming's *Quality, Productivity and Competitive Position* (1982) and A. V. Feigenbaum's *Total Quality Control* (1983), which described the use of quality control at every level of an organization. These references remain excellent sources for corporate managers interested in understanding the principles behind TQM.

Unfortunately, many American companies failed to recognize the importance of quality improvement. There were, however, some that saw the value of incorporating TQM concepts into their business and production processes. Among these were Ford Motor Company, AT&T, Hewlett-Packard, 3M, Motorola, Bridgestone Tire Company, the Xerox Corporation, Florida Power and Light, and the Commercial Nuclear Fuel Division at Westinghouse. Each of these, and others, actively sought to apply the principles of TQM advocated by Juran, Deming, and Crosby. Many of these TQM pioneers were later recognized for their achievements with the prestigious Malcolm Baldrige Quality Award.

In the federal sector, the first formal application of TQM was in the Department of Defense. Naval Air Systems Command started a quality improvement program in the early 1980s, and the Internal Revenue Service (IRS) instituted a similar effort to improve its management processes in 1985. The IRS Ogden Service Center adopted TQM in 1986.

These efforts in the federal sector, like those in Japan and American private industry, were based on the work and findings of Deming. Unlike the private sector, however, federal agencies often find themselves challenged by congressional mandates and micromanagement of their internal operations for political reasons. They also have to deal with entrenched bureaucracies, to whom delighting a customer is a totally foreign concept.

There was, however, slow and steady adoption of Deming's principles in American manufacturing during the 1980s. There was also some involvement in TQM in the service industry, to a lesser degree; but until the late 1980s there was almost no acceptance or use of these ideas in hospitals or elsewhere in the medical profession. One exception was an attempt by the Hospital Corporation of America to implement TQM principles. Perhaps the greatest impetus to adopt TQM in health care came in 1987, with the establishment of the National Demonstration Project on Quality Improvement in Health Care. This ambitious project, hosted by Harvard Community Health Plan of Massachusetts, funded by the John A. Hartford Foundation, and headed by Don Berwick, involved twenty-one health care organizations committed to incorporating, to the best of their ability, the tools of modern quality improvement into their operations. The project issued its first report in 1988, and in 1990 it published a compilation of its findings and major lessons learned (Berwick, Godfrey, & Roessner, 1990). Many of these lessons have become truisms of TQM practiced in health care settings. For example, the report warns that involving doctors is difficult and that nonclinical processes draw early attention. Ultimate success, it claims, is tied to active leadership involvement. This project and its findings have had a profound effect on the subsequent introduction of TQM principles into health care settings all over the country. By setting a standard and identifying common problems and mistakes, the project's participants and authors have given every physician and administrator a deeper understanding of the value of the total quality concept and the difficulty they will face in adopting it.

The late eighties also saw the widespread implementation of TQM concepts in both the private and the federal sectors. In 1988, Motorola won the first National Quality Award, created as a result of the Malcolm Baldrige National Quality Improvement Act of 1987. Under the auspices of this act, the secretary of the U.S. Department of Commerce and the president are authorized to confer the award on companies and other organizations that have "substantially benefitted the economic or social well-being of the United States through improvements in the quality of their goods or services resulting from the effective practice of quality management" (Garvin, 1991, p. 80). The award was dubbed the Malcolm Baldrige Quality Award after the former secretary of the Department of

Commerce. The awarding of this prize and the publicity surrounding the event galvanized many private corporations into initiating or strengthening their own efforts at quality management. The federal government was not far behind; also in 1988, an executive order called for a governmentwide program to improve the quality of government services. Under this order, each government agency was required to establish programs to improve quality and productivity by 1991.

The Office of Management and Budget (OMB), an arm of the executive branch, issued a circular that directed federal agencies to continuously improve the quality, timeliness, efficiency, and effectiveness of their products and services by implementing total quality management practices. The circular called for commencement of the process by 1991. This publication heralded the official and explicit endorsement of TQM concepts by OMB and the entire federal government.

The leadership in the Department of Veterans Affairs also recognized the need for an organized approach to the continuous improvement of medical care. In August 1990, James W. Holsinger Jr., M.D., VHA's chief medical director, signed a memorandum to all VHA employees endorsing the implementation of TQM in the organization. In November of that same year, the secretary of veterans affairs, Edward J. Derwinski, issued a formal memorandum stating, "We will come to grips, once and for all, with the fundamental question of quality. We will fulfill our moral obligation to consistently provide quality care to our patients. We will hold ourselves to the highest standards; . . . Quality is not negotiable, and [it] is . . . our primary mission. . . . We must lead the federal government in implementing Total Quality Management" (Department of Veterans Affairs internal memo, 1990).

The TQM concepts of Deming and Juran are at work in VHA facilities across the country today. This book chronicles the systemwide implementation called for by Derwinski and Holsinger. A central tenet of TQM is that quality is determined by processes, not individuals. Employees at all levels of VHA are learning to analyze processes, collect data, and convert it into useful information. They are starting to take that information and make necessary changes in the processes of caregiving to improve the quality and timeliness of the care received by their veteran patients.

There is ample evidence that health has been and is one of the fundamental concerns of humankind. People in various cultures and in almost every age have demonstrated concern about quality of life and the care needed to enhance and preserve it. Formal systems and historical luminaries have aimed to either develop or maintain an environment that produces the highest possible quality of health care. Western civilization has given considerable time and thought to the organization and effectiveness of health care delivery systems.

The development and maturation of the practice of medicine into a scientific discipline characterized by use of the scientific method and, especially recently, rapidly advancing technology has not fundamentally changed the need for proper organization and monitoring of the system to ensure timely care of the highest possible quality. In fact, the more complicated and exacting health care processes become, the greater the need for reliable systems and a means to ensure quality and efficiency.

VHA has recognized that in order to exist and thrive in the health care community of the future, quality can no longer be the delegated responsibility of quality committees or remote staff units but must become the responsibility of every employee. In this new age of health care delivery, total quality and continuous improvement in that quality will be the hallmark by which one hospital or provider differentiates itself from another. VHA has committed itself to being a leader in the field of quality health care. How this vision evolved and was applied throughout the system is told in the following chapters.

References

Berwick, D. M., Godfrey, A. B., & Roessner, J. (1990). *Curing health care: New strategies for quality improvement.* San Francisco: Jossey-Bass.

Crosby, P. B. (1979). *Quality is free: The art of making quality certain.* New York: Penguin Books.

Deming, W. E. (1982). *Quality, productivity, and competitive position.* Cambridge, MA: MIT Press.

Feigenbaum, A. V. (1983). *Total quality control.* New York: McGraw-Hill.

Garvin, D. A. (1991, November-December). How the Baldrige award really works. *Harvard Business Review,* pp. 80–93.

Juran, J. M. (Ed.). (1979). *Juran's quality control handbook*. New York: McGraw-Hill.

Relman, A. (1988). Assessment and accountability: The third revolution in medical care. *New England Journal of Medicine, 319,* 1220–1222.

Shewhart, W. (1931). *The economic control of the quality of manufactured product*. New York: McGraw-Hill.

Walton, M. (1986). *The Deming management method*. New York: Putnam.

Part Two

The Path to Total Quality Improvement

Chapter Four

Pioneers and Precursors

Robert P. Means and Joseph R. Nagel

There is an old adage that states that "we sometimes have to look backwards to see where we are going." The brief journey of the Veterans Health Administration (VHA) toward a quality-improvement environment may be perceived by some as little more than a series of fits and starts. Perhaps the various philosophies that have guided management thinking in this century, as well as the many VHA programs and experiments that have seemingly failed, should instead be seen as part of a natural evolution of management. For out of each "failed" experiment came a significant lesson, a clearer direction for the future, an incremental step toward a better tomorrow.

The contributions of numerous management philosophers and practitioners have helped guide VHA along a path toward a more participative management approach. A number of initiatives that occurred during the 1980s at VHA's predecessor, the Veterans Administration's Department of Medicine and Surgery (DM&S), are indicative of this trend.

An early attempt to introduce participative management into DM&S was the Motivational Dynamics program. In the late 1970s, the St. Louis regional medical education center (RMEC) purchased an educational course called "Motivational Dynamics" from Control Data Corporation. The course consisted of twelve modules of video- and print-based learning materials summarizing the works of past and present management theorists. Motivational Dynamics progressively exposed managers and supervisors to seminal thinking in the areas of individual, group, and organizational development.

The course was recognized by many as a fine theoretical introduction to management thinking that included as much as possible in a packaged twenty-four-hour course.

The RMEC system implemented Motivational Dynamics using a train-the-trainer format and had some limited success with it. Some hospitals delivered the course to a majority of their management and supervisory staff. In some hospitals the course was considered successful within a given service or department.

There were two criticisms of Motivational Dynamics that probably limited its success. It was recognized as a fine theoretical overview of management philosophy, but it was criticized for being deficient in suggestions for practical applications. Secondly, DM&S in general may not have been ready for Motivational Dynamics. Many hospital directors' career paths had depended on a traditional, authoritative management style, and it was difficult for them to shed this orientation in favor of a more participative approach.

Another attempt to become more participatory involved quality circles, first implemented at DM&S in 1981 as part of a pilot study. Based on the work of W. Edwards Deming and Joseph Juran, quality circles were an American idea that did not become popular in this country until the Japanese began using them and surpassing U.S. industry in virtually all productivity measures. A quality circle is composed of seven to ten workers who do the same type of work. The circle meets regularly and analyzes problems specific to their work situation. They use data and statistical methods to determine solutions and make recommendations.

As a result of successful experiences with quality circles in both the public and private sectors, in 1981 the Veterans Administration (VA) initiated a quality circles pilot program at five of its hospitals: Albany, New York; Gainesville, Florida; Phoenix, Arizona; Togus, Maine; and Knoxville, Iowa. Following the training of steering committees, facilitators, and quality circle leaders, a year-long experiment ensued. Early reports from the five pilot sites were positive: quality circles were successfully solving problems and enhancing hospital effectiveness.

Based on the success of these five pilot programs, the VA decided to expand the quality circle effort to the larger DM&S system. In July 1982, representatives from each RMEC assembled in St. Louis and were introduced to the quality circle concept.

RMEC representatives then visited VA hospitals that had expressed an interest in quality circles and oriented them to the concept, providing them with training materials and discussing implementation issues and the potential consequences of using quality circles as a management approach.

One issue that limited the success of the quality circle effort was a headquarters mandate that any hospital considering the implementation of quality circles appoint a full-time quality circle facilitator-coordinator. Many hospitals decided that they could not afford to devote a full-time executive to this effort. The headquarters official coordinating the quality circle program was convinced, however, that any attempt to implement this management philosophy required nothing less than a full-time facilitator-coordinator if it were to be at all successful.

Another issue that limited the success of the pilot program was a lawsuit filed by the American Federation of Government Employees (AFGE) union. A perceived lack of information by AFGE leadership about quality circles and their long-term effect on the management-labor relationship was the impetus for the lawsuit. During the prolonged litigation that followed, hospital leadership support for quality circles waned.

It was indeed unfortunate that the quality circle effort was not successful systemwide. In 1983 a group of DM&S staff was invited to present the results of the quality circle pilot program at an International Association of Quality Circles meeting in Memphis, Tennessee. Individuals at that meeting from other government agencies and health care institutions expressed a high degree of interest in the concept.

As progressive as the quality circle movement seemed at the time, in retrospect it was quite limited in its scope. It sought merely to have work teams engage in problem solving and process improvement rather than pursue entirely new systems or processes for doing work. In the final analysis, perhaps the VA's timing was simply off. Perhaps a traditional bureaucratic system as large and encumbered as the VA needed more time to digest this "systems approach" to management. During the early 1980s, the VA was a fairly static organization, and it probably lacked sufficient discomfort (that is, motivation) to push systemwide changes in management style within DM&S. Other events that occurred in the latter half of the 1980s got the attention of VA leadership and provided the extrinsic and intrinsic motivators to begin the process of significantly altering management practices.

In 1986 the Veterans Administration was heavily scandalized in the press with isolated but cumulatively embarrassing reports of substandard patient services and low-quality care. Within DM&S, a new guest relations training movement surfaced in an effort to improve relations with the department's customers and improve the public image of the VA as a health care provider. In the beginning this movement (called "guest relations" within DM&S) consisted mostly of vendor-prepared or consultant-driven training focused on a limited number of staff who had direct contact with patients. These events occurred at a time when the captains of U.S. industry were finally paying heed to the messages of Deming, Juran, and Crosby, the gurus of continuous quality improvement. Several individuals and organizations within the VA saw a need for a broad systems approach to improving services; such an approach was available via guest relations training. Their efforts represent the precursors of the more comprehensive total quality improvement (TQI) movement at VHA. Their stories are somewhat unique in that they started with little or no fanfare and matured to a point that greatly facilitated the start-up of a formal VHA national TQI approach in 1991. They had built a foundation upon which these concepts of continuous quality improvement could grow. While only four cases are cited here, they represent some of the most recognizable and enduring continuous quality improvement practices during this time in the VA's history.

The series of case examples presented below is essentially about people and organizations within the Department of Veterans Affairs and VHA who were willing to anticipate the future. They were innovative and willing to take risks to make life for themselves and others better. They were in a sense the pioneers that cut the path for the more timid managers who followed. In essence, they were "paradigm pioneers," interested in changing the fundamental way problems are solved. They realized that their work would require not only courage but considerable time and commitment (Barker, 1993). They may not have received the recognition of a Ray Kroc (McDonald's), Sam Walton (WalMart), or Fred Smith (Federal Express), but they possessed similar ideas, such as knowing intuitively that there was a better world they could help create, and in retrospect their efforts in health care were clearly at the cutting edge.

Looking back, much of what these brief case examples represent is a chronology of the inevitability and rapidity of change over the past decade within VHA. They also reflect the decline of the autocratic manager and the emergence of the advocate and leader for change. Today, less emphasis is placed on individual problem solving and more attention is paid to creative teamwork that contributes to whole systems improvement (Weisbord, 1991). A preoccupation with crisis management has been replaced by a more strategic emphasis on learning to anticipate the future.

Many of these stories reflect efforts on the part of individuals and organizations to embrace rather than resist changes designed to improve health care delivery and customer service. Many of these individuals and organizations continue to confront such changes at an unpredictable and relentless pace. The period of time described below represents the beginning of the end of the bureaucratic model of organizational life, a product of the industrial age, in which leaders were preoccupied with control, order, and predictability. In its place is emerging a new order of democratic, egalitarian organizations relying on teams, clusters, alliances, networks, and collaboratives flexible enough to rapidly form, reform, and disband, depending on the needs of the clients they serve (Pinchot & Pinchot, 1993). Thus has been born the collaborative organization led by individuals, groups, and teams interested in learning from one another to create a future that is responsive to customers.

What remains interesting about all these cases is that the returns on investing in TQI were all greater than anticipated. What was learned was significant enough to reduce resistance to future change efforts, and without exception, these efforts continue today in some fashion. Each case description is included to provide insights into how the effort began, what form it took, its successes and failures, what key lessons were learned, and how the pioneering effort made the transition to a more comprehensive approach to continuous improvement easier.

Case 1: Pilot Project Creates Foundation for TQI
Overview

By 1988, the early efforts within DM&S to address guest relations training requirements had proved limited in scope and were providing little more than cosmetic treatment of a much deeper concern about improving quality at all levels of the hospital. The issue was more than how to properly greet veteran patients. In fact, a more comprehensive examination of internal and external customer and supplier requirements and DM&S operational processes was needed in order to understand how to more efficiently and effectively service veterans and their beneficiaries. Working with the director of Medical District 15 and staff from the Cleveland, Ohio; Indianapolis, Indiana; Danville, Illinois; Marion, Indiana; and Fort Wayne, Indiana VA hospitals, the Cleveland RMEC served as broker for a pilot venture in quality management. Vendor-prepared packages on "total quality awareness" and "quality management skills" were introduced (by Organizational Dynamics, Inc.) to representatives from the five hospitals. The programs were designed to address the needs of patients, coworkers, managers, liaisons with other services, and many others who were both customers and suppliers in an interlocking chain of services. Meeting the collective needs of customers and suppliers, whether external (patient, family) or internal (coworker, manager), is integral to developing a quality product or service. The training programs were designed not only to raise awareness of quality in everyday work life but also to inculcate the processes necessary to maintain or enhance quality in a dramatically changing health care environment in which everyone was being asked to do more with less. Training modules included assessment, exercises, and readings on a variety of continuous improvement issues. While the initial focus was on awareness of customer and supplier relationships, the more advanced modules also addressed the creation of process improvement teams. Special training was available for managers to acquire skills in supporting a team-driven work environment.

While representatives from all five hospitals were completing the basic curriculum on total quality awareness, two distinct projects emerged. First, at Cleveland the focus of the program became guest relations training for several key services. The program was modified by an outside consultant and planning team. The consultant was subsequently hired by the hospital as an organization development expert with responsibility to expand the work of the project; the consultant did so by training trainers for work in those medical and administrative services that were interested in and receptive to this type of change process.

Second, an extensive assessment of Medical District 15 hospital needs resulted in a significant redesign of the original Organizational Dynamics, Inc., total quality awareness print material to accommodate DM&S's renewed perspective. The project also included a major conference in which key management as well as staff from each hospital participated in a session with a leading quality guru, George Labovitz, Ph.D., president of Organizational Dynamics, Inc., the key vendor. Ultimately, four out of five pilot sites became actively involved in VHA's TQI program. The pilots were successful in highlighting the future requirements of any organization wanting to be successful in implementing TQI.

Results

1. Top managers' initial response was to *consent* but not necessarily *commit* to the process. In three hospitals, the directors and members of the executive staff eventually became actively involved, some serving as team members. It was at these three hospitals that VHA's national TQI program would be successfully introduced some three years later.

2. The degree to which various levels of staff were involved also served as a barometer of success. A small core of staff at two of the four hospitals were heavily invested in modifying the original vendor package script. Their high level of involvement gave the staff a sense of empowerment, but it had two negative side effects. First, the redesign process took nearly a year to complete, and some individuals lost energy for the project. Second, having a small core staff directing this effort meant that only a limited number of persons were involved until the training was actually delivered.

3. These pilots were truly the beginning of lengthier team efforts, which were not an easy sell since people still retained the

mental model of a "quick fix" via training. Numerous issues and concerns emerged as the implementation effort proceeded. Many issues were not anticipated; some only experience would rectify, and others required additional resources and staff time. The Cleveland RMEC, serving as broker, had not anticipated all the additional requirements, which further complicated implementation.

4.   While the initial plan was to improve customer relations, particularly by providing quality services to patients after concise training interventions, early in the process it became evident that to do so required substantial shifts in attitude, behavior, and service. It meant answering fundamental questions about organizational mission, vision, values, and, as a result, organizational culture. These questions in turn raised issues of assessing the organization's current practices as well as its readiness to engage in this type of change process. On the positive side, this led to it acquiring an assessment tool that ultimately became part of VHA's national program.

5.   The location of this pilot within the functional framework of the organization also became an issue. While the process initially started with a cross-section of interested staff, questions were raised as to why it was not driven by the organization's education and training function. The project in all cases forced the hospitals to examine their education and training function, and in at least three cases out of four, there was ultimately some form of change or revitalization in the unit.

6.   During these pilot programs there were several changes in top management at three of the five hospitals. It was a tribute to those who worked to embed this process across key services that in these three hospitals the process flourished in spite of the changes in leadership.

As a result of this effort, three of the institutions joined and remained in VHA's national TQI effort. In fact, the Indianapolis hospital was recently recognized as a leader in quality management, winning the Department of Veterans Affairs Robert W. Carey Quality Award in the health care category. A fourth hospital ventured on its own into quality improvement, without support of the national program, and has made progress.

Case 2: Expanding an Approach to Quality Improvement
Overview

Quality improvement became the focus of a special initiative in the southern region in February 1988. Sparked by systemwide concern that the VA's image was being tarnished by isolated but well-publicized incidents of inferior care, the Birmingham RMEC and five VA hospitals met to design an intervention aimed at improving communications. They implemented a related guest relations program. A cross-section of staff designed the initial intervention and labeled it with the acronym IMAGES—Improving Morale and Giving Excellent Service. The outcome was a three-hour training intervention designed to improve the morale, performance, and interpersonal skills of employees throughout the organization. Emphasis was placed on universal awareness of the benefits of courtesy, respect, camaraderie, positive attitudes, and enthusiasm toward patients, their families, visitors, and fellow employees.

IMAGES was not solely a guest relations program. The planners felt they needed to produce a compelling event that would serve an ongoing purpose within their facilities. They wanted something that would create enough energy and action to change people's perceptions of their institution from that of a noncaring bureaucracy to that of a caring, quality hospital. They felt that in order to be successful the effort needed top management commitment, a clear mission and vision communicated to all employees, improved staff communication and support, and rewards and celebrations to recognize successful efforts to improve quality service. Thus, using the outline of an already successful program in a local community hospital, the planning group of mid-level managers and Birmingham RMEC staff created the IMAGES program.

One of the strengths of their work was their broad systems approach to this issue. The intent was to help VA hospitals look at the strategic rather than simply the tactical aspects of improving quality. This strategic approach was strikingly similar to VHA's national TQI implementation, which would appear four years after the start of IMAGES. The planners created an implementation strategy that required interested hospital management to involve all staff. In most cases, the RMEC conducted retreats with top management and service chiefs prior to the delivery of the IMAGES program. Four to eight facilitators from each hospital were trained on-site so they could learn the necessary concepts as they completed the local intervention. IMAGES also became a part of these hospitals' new employee orientation. Each IMAGES training session was three hours in length, multidisciplinary, and limited to thirty-five employees.

IMAGES PLUS (People Learning Unique Strategies) was a national follow-up to the initial IMAGES program. During the initial program, participants were asked to identify areas of care or service that could be targets for improvement. Subsequent programs were developed by the local facility and/or RMEC to enhance service excellence.

Results

1.   The broad systems approach, illustrated with flow diagrams, helped managers and staff visualize the need for this training and the fact that it fit into an overall system of change. It helped them appreciate what other work still needed to be done and how all these pieces fit into a whole structure of concerns related to quality improvement.

2.   The planners capitalized on the successes of another similar program and modified it to meet the VA's requirements.

3.   Hospitals in the region felt that the IMAGES program was of their own design, because they participated along with the Birmingham RMEC in its creation as well as its implementation.

4.   IMAGES was an initial assessment tool for quality improvement in the hospital.

5.   Twenty-two hospitals and four outpatient clinics were involved, and many continue to use IMAGES.

6.   The multidisciplinary approach proved effective in getting various levels of administrative as well as clinical staff to communicate and plan around quality issues.

7.   The three-hour length of the program was a manageable amount of time to allow for almost everyone's attendance.

8.   Several of the facilitators have become executive assistants or trainers for quality as part of the national VHA TQI program.

9. Completing the program gave people a better sense of their individual responsibility to improve quality care.

Lessons Learned

1. Senior management was asked to provide introductions at each training effort; when that did not occur, the impact of IMAGES seemed to be limited.

2. The program started out as voluntary but was made mandatory at most hospitals to ensure universal attendance; the result was that some staff were less attentive participants.

3. Sustaining this program over time has become an issue for some sites as facilitators move on or top management changes.

4. IMAGES PLUS, the effort to identify other quality issues, was great at getting some hospitals to develop action plans and conduct training in quality improvement beyond the initial three-hour session, but in some cases it raised but then failed to address certain expectations and needs.

The one major strength of the program was its natural assimilation with the national TQI effort that emerged in 1991. IMAGES was used by some as a kickoff to a more comprehensive TQI effort. It provided some of the initial assessment data regarding areas and processes in need of improvement, and it enabled hospital staff to focus on the foundational components of TQI by establishing mission and vision statements. IMAGES is now viewed as an option for hospitals interested in reinvesting themselves in customer relations activities in accordance with new VHA service standards.

Case 3: A Management College Drives a Quality Movement

Overview

The director of VHA Region 1, Al Washko, created the vision for a regionwide, customer-focused initiative. The program, named Service Excellence, focused on improving health care services to veterans while at the same time making the region's hospitals better places to work for all employees. This data-driven approach to improving processes and systems represented a significantly broader approach to customer relations than many of the guest relations programs of this same era.

Working with key regional staff, an outside consultant spearheaded the mass customization of education, training, and quality assessment tools that were ultimately used by three-quarters of the region's facilities. The planners used an emergent design based on inputs from selected executives, managers, supervisors, and field staff. The implementation strategy was based on the development of a "virtual management college"; region managers and executives constituted the brain trust for testing the design of programs and were responsible for conducting assessments and related training.

The program modules grew in numbers over the years, with a primary focus on customer requirements. The introductory module was routinely taught by the regional director. A series of modules were developed on various management and supervisory issues that had affected the project. These included topics such as staff selection, negotiation, positive reinforcement, and, in the final phases, tools for TQI and facilitation of groups.

Some forty managers traveled throughout the region conducting on-site training, training other managers, and offering various types of quality training that eventually reached twenty thousand employees. The program was coordinated regionally from 1988 to 1993. A testament to the success of this initiative is that the program stayed intact during a five-year time period.

Results

1. The data-driven process, which included preassessments, in-process assessments, and postassessments as well as action plans, provided information essential in measuring results and acknowledging both successes and failures.

2. The regional director and the management college faculty (facility management) served as excellent role models for employees and other managers.

3. Assessment tools were created to measure organizational culture and climate and to identify processes that ultimately served as indices of success.

4. The interventions at these facilities encouraged the creation of early versions of process action teams, which now produce positive changes in VA medical centers across the country.

5. The program created a common language around customer service, quality, and service excellence.

6. The effort represented a systems approach, examining quality issues in search of root causes.

7. The program was a catalyst for a series of follow-up training activities designed by local VA hospitals.

8. Program acceptance was significantly high, in part because each activity was based on locally derived needs.

9. The program had wide appeal because it was designed by VHA staff and focused on VHA issues.

Not surprisingly, some of the program strengths were also its weaknesses. The emergent model approach often meant lengthy delays between development of one program and its delivery regionwide. There was only a limited number of managers serving as trainers for the region, and they were only available part-time. The long-term working relationship with one consultant led to some difficulties in VHA's obtaining copyrights on certain materials and therefore restricted their distribution.

The creation of the national TQI initiative systemwide also presented a dilemma. During 1991 and 1992, the management college continued to expand program offerings to include TQI tools and group facilitation skills, to prevent the region from having to start all over again using similar approaches available via VHA's national TQI program. The task of sustaining such a comprehensive quality approach eventually led to a proposal to merge both efforts. However, the concept grew increasingly complex because of changes in the leadership and key support staff in the Region 1 office and a series of standardized requirements necessary to participate in the national pilot. Support for the management college was removed as the national initiative, driven by a flood of new resources, took hold.

Clearly the efforts of the college and its cadre of faculty laid the groundwork for many VA hospitals to readily assimilate the more comprehensive TQI approach available throughout VHA.

Case 4: Veterans Benefit Administration—
A Pilot Becomes a Model Program

Overview

In September 1988, senior managers from the VA regional office and insurance center (ROIC) in Philadelphia, inspired by the vision of their director, the late Robert W. Carey, began their continuous improvement journey by attending Dr. Joseph Juran's conference "Making Quality Happen." Their decision to attend was the result of their own conclusion that the one thousand employees in the regional office needed to improve their delivery of services to veterans, including the processing of disability compensation, pensions, education allowances, and home loan guarantees and the provision of vocational rehabilitation and counseling. With the assistance of QUALTEC, a subsidiary of Florida Power and Light Company, the ROIC approached its TQI effort by focusing on three major processes:

- *Quality improvement:* Employees were empowered through their participation in quality improvement teams. They sought to continually make small, incremental improvements in the way they did business.
- *Quality planning:* The ROIC targeted areas that were important to customers by using surveys and focus groups to identify customer needs and develop quality measurement systems based on their expectations. By merging this information with business needs, they set goals and objectives for their organizations and worked to ensure that they were realized.
- *Quality control:* The ROIC used a variety of measurement systems to evaluate performance, compare it to their goals, and act on the difference. Their ultimate goal was to do the right things right the first time.

The ROIC formed subcouncils for various sections within the center and the division's lead team to discover processes in need of improvement and implement training and support for improvement teams.

The initial strengths of these improved efforts were to enhance decision making based on customer data, not perceptions or guesswork. An overall plan for improvement was drawn up and shared with all center employees, along with a common language for improvement. Employees became involved in decision making and in setting their own performance standards. Feedback mechanisms were created so that employees were provided with continuous measures of their performance against customer standards.

The results of these efforts included the distribution of millions of dollars to veterans for benefits that had previously been unknown and gone unclaimed; creation of a toll-free 800 number for insurance policyholders and their beneficiaries; a substantial reduction in the number of congressional inquiries; reduction in claims processing times; and improvement in the quality of work life with the creation of an employee fitness center, day-care centers, flextime, an employee assistance program, and expanded health services.

These successes did not come without mistakes and regrets. Teams learned to slow down the pace of implementation. Too many teams and too many processes led to a refocusing on a vital few. It would have been better to introduce cross-functional teams later on, after team members better understood their own work processes. Management took on too much too fast, without fully understanding their new responsibilities in supporting this effort.

Lessons Learned

1. Top management has retained a definitive role in managing the organization using this team improvement process. Not all decisions are by consensus, but all are driven by customer data internal and external to the organization.

2. Employees are periodically asked to complete a quarterly self-assessment of their progress toward meeting customer requirements, to provide feedback to one another as well as to management.

3. Employees are cross-trained to learn about other aspects of a process that impacts a beneficiary.

4. Employees are recognized and honored for the work they do, and extra step increases are available as incentives to provide excellent work.

5.   Self-directed work teams continue to emerge as the process of improvement matures.

6.   Each year the entire center celebrates its successes on Groundhog Day.

Further evidence of the success of TQI has been the numerous presidential and National Performance Review prototype awards that the ROIC staff have received for their work. In 1992, the secretary of veterans affairs created the Robert W. Carey Quality Award in honor of the visionary leadership he provided the quality improvement movement in the department. A testimonial to Carey's leadership is the fact that four years after his untimely death at age 44, the ROIC continues its quality improvement journey. The award is now coveted by those VA hospitals selected each year for their efforts in creating a continuous improvement effort that supports a customer-driven culture.

Conclusion

Past experience is often the best predictor of future behavior. Even this limited number of case examples offers some insights into what the future may hold.

The 1980s and early 1990s saw a shift in management practice from a focus on the internal workings of an organization to how its products and services meet its customers' needs. Further, efficiency and effectiveness in operational processes took precedence over the traditional, functional focus. Finally, the organizational focus is no longer management-centered but employee-centered. Driven by a need to improve VHA's service, care, and image, VHA managers began to experiment with participatory forms of governance that emphasized collective employee involvement. This resulted in an increase in creative solutions and, in a few cases, an empowered workforce.

These cases represent some of the early indicators that executives can give up the notion of having to know and control everything and still lead organizations to levels of high performance and success (Schein, 1993). There are some data to suggest that when leaders are committed, become involved, and learn along with frontline workers, continuous improvement efforts have a greater chance of sustaining themselves, even when the leadership changes. VHA leaders and managers saw these efforts as opportunities to practice and model a new, more inclusive and participative style of management. For these leaders, VHA's continuous improvement initiatives were opportunities to test several new or newly configured management practices, such as the use of teams and statistical data to improve decision making. These efforts created opportunities for these leaders to expand their view of whole systems theory and renew their understanding of the consequences that decisions and actions have on the entire chain of customers and suppliers. VHA leaders' point of view is no longer focused solely on issues within functional units but horizontally across their entire organization; consequently, their decisions are more valuable and beneficial to everyone.

For staff, these initiatives represented emancipation from a colonial, paternalistic form of governance to one that was, at least at some level, more democratic and empowering. Every case described here included an effort to involve staff in the planning, design, and implementation of TQI processes. This was a particularly powerful approach when staff were given the opportunity to lead efforts, whether as trainers or leaders of process improvement teams. Their sense of importance and worth was further enhanced when they were asked to serve on quality councils or similar groups along with executives, managers, and key institutional decision makers.

To a certain degree all these efforts represented a beginning of fundamental, not just incremental, cultural change. Efforts to establish a mission, a vision, and value statements may have been more symbolic than substantive, but they offered a beginning point for VHA organizations to look where they were headed strategically, not just tactically. Each effort led to discussions (if not actions) about how to make structures and functions within VHA organizations more customer-friendly and more capable of producing quality products and services. Teams, councils, and networks represented but a few of these forums. Ultimately each organization's commitment to look to the long term helped erode criticism of these efforts as the "latest management fad." This longer journey meant greater resource requirements, but it often provided convincing evidence that the organization's commitment to this new type of work was real.

These cases offered many valuable lessons (not the least of which was an awareness of conditions that hampered the likelihood of success):

1.   There is a significant advantage to having leaders demonstrate commitment through actual involvement in change efforts. Consenting to this type of work is the first indication that management wants others to change.

2.   Leaders' and managers' fears and anxiety about losing power and control to an empowered workforce can sabotage the best of intentions. Major efforts are needed to define managers' role in this process and, where appropriate, provide them with new skills.

3.   Leaders and managers are interested in doing everything. Too much, too fast was a typical response, and it led in some cases to lack of resources and time to accomplish all the work.

4.   Teams are more often successful when care is given to membership selection and training.

5.   Consultants are often inappropriate for the VHA environment, and vendor-prepared materials are often incomplete. Suitably modified packages can play a significant part in individual and team learning, but there is a point at which they can burden staff and delay implementation.

6.   Training often can become the focus of the process, when it only represents one part of a successful effort. In the cases examined above, numbers of staff trained did not necessarily equate with a changed culture or better service to clients.

7.   The most difficult work is not starting the process but sustaining the effort. In three cases the primary task was to assimilate local efforts into VHA's national TQI effort.

References

Barker, J. A. (1993). *Paradigms: The business of discovering the future*. New York: HarperCollins.

Pinchot, G., & Pinchot, E. (1993). *The end of bureaucracy and the rise of the intelligent organization*. San Francisco: Berrett-Koehler.

Schein, E. H. (1993). How can organizations learn faster? The challenge of entering the green room. *Sloan Management Review, 34*(2).

Weisbord, M. R. (1991). *Productive workplaces: Organizing and managing for dignity, meaning, and community*. San Francisco: Jossey-Bass.

Chapter Five

A Starting Point: Hines VA Hospital

Larry Malby with John R. Fears

The question of why the Veterans Health Administration (VHA) embraced total quality improvement (TQI) does not yield a simple answer. One could dismiss the advent of TQI in VHA as a simple reaction to forces under way throughout private industry and government. In the early 1990s, thousands of people in almost all government departments and agencies were engaged in the pursuit of TQI in numerous forms and shapes, and those activities have continued to evolve (Federal Quality Institute, 1995). In fact, with the advent of the Reinventing Government movement in the early days of the Clinton-Gore administration, it was difficult for any government entity to avoid at least paying lip service to some aspects of TQI. Because of the governmentwide fascination with TQI, some would say that it was inevitable that VHA would eventually begin to implement TQI principles. Inevitable or not, VHA did embark on a TQI journey. Previous chapters showed how the Veterans Administration (VA) health care system evolved, and provided evidence of early strivings for the kind of team- and customer-focused activity that presaged TQI. This chapter will examine the TQI journey from the perspective of VHA headquarters, describing how the journey started and some of the major and minor obstacles that plagued its early days.

When one looks at the triggering events, the adoption of TQI in VHA does not look at all inevitable; instead, it looks almost accidental, at least in terms of its timing. Hindsight shows that early

events and characters came together almost fortuitously to shape
the systemwide pursuit of excellence that is now called TQI in
VHA. As with any story, one must select a starting point. In this
case, it dates back to the summer of 1988, when Organizational Dynamics, Inc., a nationally known consulting firm, sent out invitations to attend a seminar on management training. One of these
invitations was sent to VHA headquarters in Washington, D.C.
Since the invitations involved "training," those who minded the
mail for VHA (then called the Department of Medicine and
Surgery, or DM&S) dutifully routed it to the Office of Management
Support, which was headed by Charles V. "Chuck" Yarbrough. He
selected his chief of executive development, Patricia Hicks, along
with an organizational development expert, Susan Blount, to attend. What these two persons saw at that seminar was a demonstration of the potential of TQI. Hicks recalled, "I vividly remember
us leaving the consultant and excitedly exclaiming all the way back
to the office, 'What if . . . what if . . . what if . . .' It seemed so impossible to dream of TQI in a government office, but the concept
was so attractive that we simply couldn't dismiss the notion. It was
not out of the realm of possibilities." They reported what they had
seen to Yarbrough, and he organized a think tank with Hicks and
Blount as members. Other VHA members of the original think
tank were Becky Hucks, Susanne Mardres, and Lynn Shepard; an
executive at the Federal Quality Institute (FQI) was also a participant. From a historical perspective, TQI in VHA is equated with
names like Holsinger, Fears, and Barbour—not Yarbrough; but
Yarbrough's establishment of the total quality think tank was the
first formal step in VHA's TQI journey.

Subsequent meetings focused on how to begin the implementation of TQI on a national basis. Given the size and complexity of
the VHA health care system, the task was formidable. By the fall of
1988, the members had formulated a basic strategy that limited the
task and reduced its initial complexity to something doable: first
engage the senior management at VHA headquarters. To that end,
they developed a plan that called for a one-hour overview of TQI
principles for key staff and a one-day TQI awareness session for
twenty-five senior managers. Yarbrough forwarded a proposal in
November 1988 to the late John A. Gronvall, then chief medical

director. As it turned out, Gronvall had been aware of the seminal work done by Donald Berwick in the National Demonstration Project. He immediately saw the proposal's potential for the VHA health care system and approved the plan. Had Gronvall not seen that potential or not been willing to act on it, VHA's TQI initiative might have stopped there.

In January 1989, the director of FQI presented a one-hour overview of TQI to key staff. This was followed in August 1989 by a one-day TQI awareness session for senior management. VHA had taken its first steps toward implementing TQI. The journey lasted about a week! It was stopped by a major obstacle—a reorganization.

For some time, Edward Derwinski, secretary of veterans affairs, had been examining the organizational structure of VHA with a view toward making it more efficient and responsive. In August 1989 he launched a major reorganization effort that consumed the energies of the organization for months. The Management Support Office was a key player in planning the reorganization, and there was no "room on the plate" for the fledgling TQI effort. The reorganization focused on restructuring VHA's seven regional offices, which exercised operational control over the VA hospitals and the twenty-eight medical districts that coordinated services among small geographic clusters of these hospitals. The reorganization reduced the seven regional offices to four and abolished the medical districts. On June 25, 1990, Congress approved Derwinsky's plan, and the ensuing months were taken up with the logistics of implementing the new organizational structure. During this time, especially during the planning phase of the reorganization, TQI faded into the background. It did not disappear, however, because the members of the think tank continued to meet.

In May 1990 an event took place that at the time appeared relatively unimportant but in retrospect had a significant influence on the future shape of TQI in VHA. The members of the think tank heard about a TQI initiative that was being pursued at the Hines VA hospital in Chicago, and they sent Patricia Hicks there to meet with the director, John Fears, and observe the program. What she saw at Hines subsequently became the prototype for a systemwide implementation of TQI. In a fairly lengthy vignette, Fears explains why and how he implemented TQI at the Hines

Hospital. His explanation shows in microcosm the essential rationale and framework for the subsequent rollout of TQI throughout the VHA health care system:

> In 1987, as the Chief Executive Officer of the Edward Hines, Jr., VA hospital in Chicago, Illinois, I found myself becoming increasingly frustrated at management's inability to "change with the times" in the face of rapid change and increased complexity in medical care. Health care had become the most complicated business in the country, and it was the largest as evidenced by the fact that it consumed 10 percent (then) of the gross national product. Work loads were increasing as people became more aware of what services were available and more demanding of their physicians and the facilities they were using.
>
> The increased complexity, which was driven by technological advances, challenged our ability to manage. Hospitals are marvels of technology. They are high-rise wonders designed to provide the caregiver (note: not the care receiver) every convenience possible. Oxygen, suction, and other highly sophisticated devices are available at the bedside. The beds themselves electronically shape themselves for comfort and ease of caregiving. Chemically treated hot water is available instantly at the tap. The floors, walls and beds are antiseptically cleaned daily. The air coming in and out of the buildings is precisely regulated to prevent the spread of infection. A generating station capable of providing power to a small town is available immediately upon loss of external power.
>
> The customers who come to the hospital, the patients, are unique. They are hurting physically or mentally as they walk through the doors, and this combination of uniqueness and pain creates an immediate challenge for any caregiver. Many have problems that are not pleasant to deal with. Patients with psychotic behavior, alcohol and drug withdrawal symptoms, and inadequate social backgrounds, including the homeless with poor hygiene, are daily visitors to admitting areas. The family members who often accompany patients also demand attention. Their expectations have grown as the sophistication of medical technology has grown.
>
> The staff required to operate a hospital are extremely diverse. They come from all levels of society. Every culture, religion, color, ethnic group, education level, and nationality is represented in a health care setting. All have different needs and expectations. Personnel administration with this much diversity is a formidable task.

Our frustration was rooted in VA's traditional management approach. In 1987, Hines was a highly structured, top level–driven system consisting of many Services (VHA hospital "Services" are normally called "departments" in non-VHA settings). It had the usual complement of 25–30 Services, such as Building Management, Engineering, Supply, Fiscal, Pharmacy, Diagnostic Radiology, Therapeutic Radiology, Medicine, Surgery, etc. Each Service had a chief who was responsible for everything done in his or her area. Coordination was accomplished through orchestrations by top management and an informal cross-function network which had evolved over the years. Manuals and policies that had been written over the past 55 years gave direction to each area. These manuals came from a highly centralized system, and in most cases were written by a person(s) far removed from the front line. Managers almost always were developed from the services in which they worked. They were selected in most cases by demonstrated ability to follow the manuals and were rewarded by how well they did the work prescribed therein.

As our frustration with the traditional management approach rose, we tried some non-traditional approaches. One of the first of these was "Hines Care." Hines Care was a team approach to management. It was designed to encourage all employees to care about the patient "customer" and to care about themselves. We conducted various activities and provided awards to encourage a more caring attitude. We believed that if we could improve our image to the patient, improve our self-image, and improve our public image, everything would get better and our overall performance would improve. The program ran about a year. Initially, it was very popular with the staff, and *it was a complete failure.*

The reason for our failure became apparent in early 1989 during a seminar conducted by the American College of Health Care Executives. The topic for the seminar was "Quality in Health Care and Pursuit of Excellence." Two of the faculty were particularly enlightening—Dr. Donald Berwick and Mr. Jack Grayson. Dr. Berwick, who has since become a leader in the TQI process in health care, gave a presentation on an article he had authored for the *New England Journal of Medicine* in which he pointed out the difference between quality *assurance* and quality *management* programs. Mr. Grayson gave an excellent presentation on the reasons for TQI and how such programs could be implemented. The seminar had been so well done that it became immediately apparent why the Hines Care program not only didn't succeed but didn't even have a chance to succeed. We had "turned our employees on" to quality and customer satisfaction but had not given them the *tools* they needed to improve performance.

That seminar was the beginning of TQI at Hines. The first step was to bring in an outside consultant to evaluate our problems and to give us some ideas about how to proceed in fostering a TQI culture. Mr. Grayson had founded an organization called the American Productivity and Quality Center (APQC); hence, it was natural to begin the journey there. Mr. Don McAdams, a Senior Consultant from APQC, visited Hines and helped us begin our quality journey.

Like many revolutions, this one had a difficult beginning. First, federal rules and regulations did not permit VHA medical facilities to obtain the services of a consultant without approval of VHA Central Office in Washington, DC, and it was known that such approval was difficult to obtain. An innovative Supply Officer at Hines came up with a solution that allowed us to use McAdams as a "lecturer" for educational purposes. He "lectured" top management for a day, and the result was a decision for Hines to become one of the first hospitals in the nation to try the TQI process. At that time, most of the TQI activity was confined to the industrial sector, and there were few guidelines for the service sector, and especially one as complicated as a hospital.

Hines began by educating 30 key people about quality management. One-half of the participants were administrative personnel, and the other half were clinical staff with about 10 physicians represented. The group was initially hesitant about the TQI process because the failure of Hines Care was fresh in their minds, but by the end of the day, everyone was at least "verbally" on board. It was obvious from the onset that the physicians harbored a "wait and see" attitude toward TQI. They had been working with the traditional quality assurance (QA) program for so many years that any new "quality" approach was thought to be duplicative in nature and would only cause more work. Also, their experiences with QA were not good, and to go from a two-letter (QA) approach to a three-letter (TQI) approach to quality did not make sense to them at the time. During the initial phase, therefore, the physicians were kept informed and involved, but they did not participate in any of the initial teams.

The organization of TQI [efforts] at Hines mirrored those that are common today. A quality leadership team (QLT) chaired by the Director led the effort. This group, in addition to giving overall leadership to the effort, was responsible for improving four major weaknesses identified in the organization: communications, data and information, rewards and recognition, and education. Four members of the QLT chaired teams to improve quality in each of these areas. The QLT also supervised the services who were responsible for efforts at their level. Each service was to have its own version of the QLT to spread TQI throughout the facility.

It quickly became obvious to everyone that training was the key function to successful implementation of TQI. With the guidance of the consultant, the QLT set up training programs that were divided into two levels. The first was an effort designed to familiarize all employees with the effort. This basic orientation to TQI was designed to ensure that employees at all levels would know the management philosophy and mission of the organization. Implementing this training was difficult and not particularly well done. Because a hospital is a 24-hour a day, 365-day a year operation, it was difficult to find the time to schedule quality orientation for everyone, particularly those on the evening and night shifts. But some training did occur and Hines had begun its TQI journey. The second phase of training was at the team level after the teams had been selected. This training consisted of team training, process training, and simple statistical tools. This education process was conducted by APQC training staff, who developed a program especially for Hines. It was a good basic program with the potential of being developed into a solid, expandable program in the future.

The first stages of this effort lasted about six months with the usual mix of successes and failures. Hines attempted to build on the successes and learn from the failures. Dietetic Service was our biggest success. Their teams completed training quickly, analyzed their processes, and came up with action plans. They implemented their plans and demonstrated remarkable improvement. For example, they improved the quality of "between meal" nourishments while reducing costs by $16,000 annually. They developed new menus for the nursing home patients and raised their level of satisfaction, and they increased the efficiency of food tray delivery and return by 25 percent. Other services did not do as well, and six months after the kickoff were still trying to get started. The fact that some succeeded and others failed can be attributed to at least five factors, several of which today have become truisms of TQI implementation.

Lessons Learned at Hines

Leadership

Carol Hall, Chief of Dietetic Service, quickly understood and believed in the process. She was not threatened, as others were, with the perceived loss of power or control. She committed her time and made sure her staff could participate fully to ensure success. She listened, learned, committed herself, and practiced TQI principles; and as a result [she] managed the best service in the hospital.

Just-in-Time Training

In some cases, training was conducted too far in advance of team activation. Whole services were given detailed training, with only a select few entering into the process. This frustrated employees who were interested in the process but not selected to serve on a team, and they started losing interest or forgot what they had learned.

Pick Low-Hanging Fruit

In several cases, we tried to do too much too fast, and frustration levels rose at the lack of success. The lesson was simple: there are hundreds of small, manageable processes in a hospital that can be studied and improved quickly. Start with these, not the complex issues, and learn from them, thus building confidence and gaining experience.

Teams Should Consist of the Players

In some of the first teams formed, there were too many levels of staff involved. The teams that were successful were those whose members actually worked in the process being studied.

Empowerment

Team members must understand and believe that if they come up with an acceptable action, they are empowered to try out the necessary changes. Too many say TQI is a glorified suggestion program where management would dissect and permit implementation if they felt like it. The teams that were successful started changes before they got "permission," based on the old adage that it is better to ask forgiveness than permission [J. R. Fears, personal communication, 1995].

Hicks returned to VHA headquarters with an appreciation of the power of TQI and of the steps needed to implement it. That visit had two major consequences for TQI at VHA. First, Fears learned about the interest at VHA headquarters for implementing TQI systemwide and the fact that Gronvall had approved it. Second, Hicks was able to observe firsthand a TQI program in operation at a VA hospital. She observed that "at Hines, I was able to see in person something that we had only been able to speculate about—TQI actually working in a VA hospital." She saw a model of implementation that could be replicated in other VA hospitals. The think tank began exploring the possibility of launching a major TQI training effort systemwide, but two obstacles loomed: first, a new management team recruited by Derwinski was taking over VHA headquarters, and second, the cost was prohibitive. Many of the senior managers who had attended the FQI training had left and been replaced by new people. But Yarbrough stayed, and the think tank stayed alive. The cost issue would not be solved until Fears arrived in VHA headquarters.

In any story of organizational change, there are pivotal events one can point to that changed the direction of the change effort. For TQI at VHA, the appointment of James W. Holsinger, Jr. M.D., as chief medical director in the summer of 1990 was such an event. Holsinger had been the director of the VA hospital in Richmond, Virginia. He was not a known advocate of TQI per se, but he brought to the office of chief medical director a management style that personified the kind of leadership needed to foster a TQI environment. His basic approach to management was collegial, emphasizing teamwork and collaboration. His management style was the fertile ground needed for the TQI philosophy to grow and flourish in VHA.

Equally important were two people Holsinger selected for his management team: John Fears and Galen Barbour, M.D. These two will always be linked with TQI in VHA. Fears was brought into VHA headquarters and assigned to head up the Office of Resource Management. He was a highly respected VA medical center director, and he brought an extensive background in VA hospital administration to VHA headquarters. Most importantly, he brought his commitment to the TQI management philosophy he had implemented at Hines and a desire to promulgate that philosophy throughout the VA health care system. Fears commented, "About six months after the implementation of the program, I left Hines, and new leadership took over. The new director continued with the TQI effort, and it has continued to grow and develop. I moved into VHA headquarters in Washington, D.C., and took many of the ideas generated by the Hines experiment with me. I had the pleasure of seeing many of these ideas and lessons implemented throughout the VA health care system, but that is a story left to others to describe."

In fact, he made the goal of implementing TQI systemwide a condition of his acceptance of a headquarters position. He explains that "when Jim Holsinger approached me about joining his management team, one of the things I told him was that I wanted to see TQI implemented throughout VHA and that I wanted to coordinate it. Jim agreed to let me do it."

Barbour was a little-known chief of medicine at the VA hospital in Hampton, Virginia, but he nonetheless had caught the eye of Holsinger. He was brought in to head up the newly created Office of Quality Management. The functions of this office had previously been performed in another part of the organization, but Holsinger was determined to confront persistent criticisms of VA health care quality, and he established this new office with an associate chief medical director reporting directly to him. The office was responsible for what health care practitioners back then called "quality assurance." But *traditional* quality assurance was not on Barbour's agenda: "Barbour recognized that traditional quality assurance activities were perceived as somewhat punitive and did not account for substantive improvements in patient care. He set about re-directing these activities from an assurance to an improvement focus" (Malby, 1994, p. 3). Barbour's focus on continuous improvement as the goal of the new Office of Quality

Management meshed nicely with Fears's view of TQI as a management philosophy.

Once again, a fortuitous set of circumstances had intervened to reestablish VHA's TQI journey. It was the merging of these three quite different but complementary personalities that allowed TQI to take root and flourish in VHA. Holsinger was the facilitator. He used the power of his office to support the TQI effort, but he left the implementation to Fears and Barbour. Fears's vision was of a TQI rollout for the entire VA health care system, modeled after the Hines experience. That model was built on the need for both TQI consulting services and training, neither of which existed in VHA on the scale needed. He brought Patricia Hicks on as his executive assistant, and the two of them engineered a massive rollout that called for consulting support and training for the two hundred thousand persons who staffed VHA's medical facilities. In his role as head of resource management, Fears was able to guide the project through the competition for resources at VHA headquarters and obtain funding to create a cadre of internal VHA trainers and for private consulting support. (The plan and the resources required to implement it are described in detail in Chapter Six.)

Barbour's vision was to change a system that ensured quality by retrospectively reviewing medical care and then "pointing the finger" at those who did not measure up to one that continuously improved quality. He brought a much-needed focus on patient care to the TQI rollout. He also recognized that physician "buy-in" was critical to successful implementation of TQI, and he was instrumental in helping to organize a group of physicians to be trained in TQI principles and then pass that training on to physicians at individual VA hospitals.

The early days of the Holsinger administration, in the summer of 1990, were filled with TQI planning. The think tank was gradually replaced by an organized TQI structure in VHA headquarters called the TQI Coordinating Committee. A full-time TQI coordinator position was eventually added in the Office of Resource Management. The TQI Coordinating Committee planned a TQI rollout for the entire VA health care system, and in a televised address on November 7, 1990, Holsinger broadcast his TQI message to the entire system. He challenged every employee with this statement: "It will be our legacy that when we enter the twenty-first century, we will be the international model for comprehensive, high-quality, efficient health care services. . . . This is, I know, an ambitious goal. Some may even say it is too much. I agree it is ambitious, but I believe it's a goal we collectively have the talent to achieve. I also believe it is a goal we must achieve for the future viability of our health care system. The means by which I believe we can accomplish our goal is through the incorporation of the concepts, programs, and practices of total quality improvement" (VHA National Satellite Broadcast, November 1990).

There it was for the first time in VHA: the philosophy of TQI would be the engine that would drive the VA health care system into the twenty-first century. It was heady stuff for the proponents of TQI, but grand pronouncements could not overcome a significant obstacle that shortly arose involving contracting for TQI consultants.

In all the excitement of creating plans and getting them approved, the TQI enthusiasts got too far out in front of mundane but necessary processes like contracting for consulting services. Nothing just happens in a bureaucracy, and the planners encountered numerous obstacles when they attempted to negotiate all of the intricacies involved in contracting for private TQI consulting support. A linchpin of the plan to implement TQI was the use of private consultants to jump-start the process until in-house VHA staff could take over this role. It took months to iron out the myriad details. Consulting firms had to be identified. Finding consulting firms with health care experience in TQI was especially challenging. Initially, planners believed they could simply select a firm listed in the *Federal Supply Schedule*. Contracting specialists quickly intervened and insisted (correctly) that all of the required steps in a competitive bidding process be followed, which can take months. Creating "specifications" and "deliverables" consumed days. The staff had to put out requests for bids, allow time for consulting firms to respond, and review and rate the applications. Then, when an application was selected, someone would enter a protest, and they had to start over again. Eventually, the contracting problems were resolved and the rollout proceeded, but only after implementation had been delayed for eight months.

The initial planning for a systemwide rollout of TQI training was eventually completed, a private consulting firm was hired, physicians who would serve as "physician consultants" were identified, and VHA staff who would be trained as "master trainers" in TQI were in place. VHA was ready to begin the process of implementing TQI systemwide. After months of hard work, a TQI consultant arrived at the Indianapolis VA hospital on August 12, 1991. If one wants to pick the date that the sun actually rose over the extended dawn of TQI in VHA, it would be that August 12 morning when that TQI consultant walked through the front doors of the Indianapolis hospital—over three years since Patricia Hicks and Susan Blount walked away from their meeting with Organizational Dynamics with a profound hope for the future. However, several obstacles arose that threatened the rollout.

One obstacle that surfaced during the planning phase involved a legitimate concern of the American Federation of Government Employees (AFGE) union. AFGE objected to the implementation of TQI because they saw it as usurping some of their traditional prerogatives. For example, they saw in the TQI principle of empowerment a threat to their traditional role of representing union employees with management. Their logic, which was quite straightforward, went like this: an empowered employee is sanctioned by management to become directly involved in management's decision-making processes; an empowered staff does not need an intermediary such as a union; therefore, there is no need for union involvement. Not surprisingly, AFGE would not accept such a conclusion.

AFGE filed an Unfair Labor Practice (ULP) complaint against VHA with the Federal Labor Relations Authority on December 3, 1990 (shortly after the November 7 satellite broadcast). A ULP is a formal charge that alleges a violation of labor-relations law. Resolving a ULP can involve a formal, legal process complete with hearings, sworn testimony, and so on, and the outcomes are legally binding. This ULP was a direct threat to VHA's systemwide TQI rollout because part of the relief demanded by AFGE was a complete cessation of TQI activity. The ULP demanded that TQI be stopped based on the contention that VHA had established a national program that affected working conditions of employees without first bargaining with the national union. If it were found that

VHA had established a national program, then by the rules of collective bargaining, VHA could have been required to stop TQI and bargain with the national union. It was also a threat because it prevented VHA headquarters from exercising appropriate control over the TQI rollout. VHA maintained throughout the disagreement that it had not "directed" TQI implementation, because the program was voluntary; rather, VHA's role was to "permit" and endorse TQI. For that reason no directives were issued by VHA concerning TQI, because a directive from headquarters would have been evidence of a nationally directed program.

As the ULP followed the requisite legal machinations, the national AFGE discouraged local unions from participating in TQI activities. In a February 8, 1991, resolution, the AFGE National Executive Council cautioned against participating in TQI, and the National Veterans Affairs Council of the AFGE continually urged local hospital unions to resist TQI. Because of the AFGE actions, many union members at VA hospitals were precluded from participating in TQI, and their lack of participation created serious compromises in the effectiveness of TQI at some hospitals. For example, at the Danville, Illinois, VA hospital, only management staff participated in early TQI training and other TQI activities. Margaret Crabb, executive assistant for TQI at Danville, stated, "Because of union objections, bargaining unit employees were not included in the initial assessment or process action team efforts, and it is almost impossible to identify a process in a VA hospital that doesn't involve some bargaining unit employees." Others were able to work out amicable solutions at the local level. For example, at the Big Spring, Texas, VA hospital, the local AFGE president, Kenneth Dodds, initially objected to TQI. In a letter to the director he stated, "I ask that you cease and desist with the . . . TQM/TQI program in its entirety until negotiations . . . are completed" (internal letter, 1992). In this case Dodds and the director were able to negotiate an amicable solution that met the local union's demands.

The effect on the headquarters TQI operation was substantial. VHA had always maintained that the TQI process was voluntary and therefore not "directed." However, the existence of a national contract for consulting services (described in Chapter Six) was perceived by some as evidence of a national program. To remove that perception, VHA agreed at one point to completely decentralize the TQI process. VHA would not contract centrally for additional consulting services but would send funds allocated for that purpose to individual hospitals. The TQI Coordinating Committee was moved out of the headquarters Office of Resource Management to the field and placed under the auspices of a committee that governed the regional medical education centers. These efforts did not resolve the issue for the Labor Relations Authority, however, and the legal machinery ground forward. It was not until Jesse Brown, the new secretary of veterans affairs (beginning in February 1992), intervened with Alma Lee, AFGE president of the National VA Council, and brought the parties together that substantive progress was made.

VHA proceeded with its TQI rollout, but not without the continual threat of stoppage. The issue was finally settled in an amicable agreement. On April 14, 1994, almost three and one-half years after the original ULP was filed, Brown and Lee signed a VA Quality Council Charter for Total Quality Improvement. This charter established the ground rules for cooperation between AFGE and VA on implementation of TQI. Once that charter was signed, the ULP was dissolved, and with it the threat to end TQI in VHA.

Finally, all VHA staff were freed up to participate in TQI. The cost of their nonparticipation while the ULP was being settled, in terms of inefficient use of consulting and training time along with the need to now provide additional training, is difficult to measure. The cost in terms of having to avoid improving processes that required bargaining unit employees and to tailor improvement activities to fit only those staff who could participate is also difficult to measure. The lesson here is obvious: *thoroughly* evaluate the implications of union involvement *before* embarking on a major change process in an organization.

Another extremely troublesome issue emerged as soon as the TQI rollout was launched. It involved the linkage between TQI and the traditional quality assurance activities that had existed in VA hospitals for years. The TQI planners simply did not appreciate the relevance of this issue—not because they ignored it but because it had so many ramifications for the deeply embedded culture of the VA health care system. What the VHA learned here should not be ignored by any health care organization that attempts to implement the principles of TQI. Others would also caution health care organizations about this issue later (Gaucher & Coffey, 1993, pp. 54–77).

Hindsight again allows us to see what happened clearly. The first hint of a problem was shown in the experience at Hines, when Fears noted that physicians' experiences with quality assurance "were not good." It is a fact that quality assurance activities in some organizations were perceived as punitive, and clinicians in those institutions would naturally resist involvement with anything associated with it. Second, the emerging role of the executive assistant for TQI called for a staff position linked to the director. Many of the executive assistants for TQI did not understand the roles and functions of the quality assurance staff, most of whom were clinicians. On the other hand, the traditional quality assurance professionals saw the attention and resources being devoted to TQI and were upset because they perceived themselves as being left out. Watching the TQI efforts proceed was especially galling to an emerging number of quality assurance professionals who had embraced the continuous improvement model propounded by Barbour, a model that was entirely consistent with TQI principles. These professionals saw themselves in the mainstream of TQI and were embittered as they saw the TQI process unfold around them but without their involvement. Finally, the private consultants did not have extensive backgrounds in health care. Most of their experiences came from the industrial and service sectors, and as a result, their activities in the initial TQI sites tended to focus on administrative issues as opposed to patient care issues. An extreme version of this "bias" came from an unnamed consultant who was alleged to have said to a group of VHA physicians, "You know health care; we know quality."

There were exceptions to this trend. For example, the Albany, New York, VA hospital, one of the first TQI sites, integrated its TQI and quality management activities from the outset. Mary Ellen Piché, executive assistant for TQI at Albany and one of the architects of that integration, observed, "We set out from the beginning with the intent to link TQI and QM [quality management]. It seemed natural, and I couldn't imagine doing it another way." Albany even changed the name from TQI to CQI (continuous quality improvement) to emphasize the linkage. But Albany was an exception.

Because the TQI rollout was under way and the consulting teams were at work, an early strategic decision was made to focus on the TQI rollout first and the linkage with quality management (QM) second. Completing the TQI overlay was the first priority. What emerged in many VA hospitals was something akin to a schism between TQI and QM. On the one hand, there was a TQI overlay that focused largely on administrative issues; on the other hand, there was the patient-focused QM infrastructure. In some cases, there was little interaction between the two. The issue was becoming sufficiently troublesome that it was placed on the agenda of the first TQI plenary session, held for the initial TQI sites in Reno in February 1992. One entire workshop addressed the issue of the interface of TQI and QM. Specific goals of that workshop included the following:

Identify necessary linkages between TQI and QM.

Discuss changes in JCAHO requirements.

Recommend approaches.

Identify support activities.

[Veterans Health Administration, 1992]

But one workshop could do little to bridge a divide so deeply embedded in the VA health care culture—the old cliche about "the horse being out of the barn" applied to this issue. Gradually (and largely imperceptibly at the time), however, change was taking place. As outside consultants became more familiar with VA hospitals, they began to recognize the need for linkage between TQI and QM. Training materials were improved by including specific examples of linkage. As VHA master trainers assumed a larger proportion of the training load, they began to use their experiences in the VA health care system. Many quality managers began to assume roles as executive assistants for TQI, bringing their knowledge directly to the TQI process. From the headquarters perspective, however, vestiges of the schism would always exist as long as the responsibilities for TQI and QM were in different offices. Thus in early 1994, the responsibility for TQI was passed to the Office of Quality Management. One of the first steps taken was to write a directive to all VA hospitals that addressed the issue of linking TQI with QM. (Such a directive was now possible because of the settlement with AFGE.) This directive, more than anything else, symbolized the end of a schism that had plagued the TQI rollout for years. The directive stated, "VHA will encourage the close integration and linkage of TQI and QM activities as a key feature in every medical facility's performance improvement activities. Appropriate linkages should be directed by and fully endorsed by the medical facility leadership. The individual medical facilities will determine the appropriate organizational structure necessary to achieve this integration and linkage" (Veterans Health Administration, 1994).

Other obstacles arose during the implementation of TQI in VA hospitals. Many of these centered around the tremendous difficulties inherent in the need to train two hundred thousand staff in the principles of TQI. But that issue is the subject of other chapters in this book.

References

Federal Quality Institute. (1995, July 31–August 3). *Proceedings of the eighth annual national conference on federal quality*. Washington, D.C.: Author.

Gaucher, E., & Coffey, R. J. (1993). *Total quality in healthcare: From theory to practice*. San Francisco: Jossey-Bass.

Malby, L. (1994, August). Linking TQI with QM in VHA. *Alliance for CME Almanac*, pp. 1–3.

Veterans Health Administration. (1992). *Proceedings of plenary session I, Reno, Nevada, February 24–26, 1992*. Washington, D.C.: Author.

Veterans Health Administration (1994, June 29). *Linking total quality improvement (TQI) with traditional quality management activity to achieve comprehensive performance improvement*. (VHA Directive 10–94–005). Washington, D.C.: Author.

Chapter Six

Rolling Out the Plan

Lynn D. Ward with Jack R. Sklar

Implementing total quality improvement (TQI) in the Veterans Health Administration (VHA) was extremely challenging primarily because there were few organizations to follow as models. While the principles of TQI have been used successfully by many manufacturing groups in the private sector and by the U.S. military, they had not been used extensively in the health care industry, in nonmilitary government organizations, or in large national organizations. VHA combines all three; namely, it is a large national government health care organization comprising nearly five hundred hospitals and outpatient clinics with over two hundred thousand employees.

Practitioners of the principles of TQI often talk about a cultural transformation that must occur in an organization for successful TQI implementation. By that they mean a fundamental change in the way an organization goes about its business each day, a change in the way its "customers" are seen, and a change in the organizational structures required to support a focus on improvement. From the beginning, it was clear that changing VHA's culture would have to involve every employee at every level. Likewise, leaders at every level would need to accept the principles of TQI as their preferred way of doing business. In the vernacular of total quality, leaders would have to "walk the talk."

A typical approach to implementing TQI in private industrial organizations has been to use external consultants to work face-to-face with leaders and employees over an extended period of time (at least a year for an effective start-up and several more years for complete implementation). This was the formula used by such well-known total quality proponents as IBM and Motorola. The relatively few experiences in VA hospitals that experimented with total quality generally followed this approach. For example, the experience at the Hines VA hospital (discussed in Chapter Five) showed that they needed at least one hundred days of external consulting services over the first year and a significant amount in the subsequent year. When VHA planners extrapolated that experience to the entire VA health care system, they determined a need for about twenty thousand consulting days, at a cost of about $30 million, to cover just one year of initial start-up. Training materials and assessment tools drove this estimated cost still higher.

Such an expense was unthinkable in VHA's fiscal environment. Thus, matching the need with the available dollars was a major challenge early on. TQI planners had to find a cheaper approach. They started by issuing a "request for proposals," or RFP (government-speak for a paper that lists requirements and requests companies to submit a bid). The RFP asked consulting firms to explain how they would roll out total quality in VA hospitals and also how they would design a multiyear plan, given the limited funding available.

A committee composed of headquarters and field staff and chaired by John Fears, the associate chief medical director for resource management, developed the framework for the RFP. This committee defined the overall approach for implementing total quality capability throughout the VHA health care system. They selected the American Productivity and Quality Center (APQC) from the six firms that responded to the bid request. APQC, based in Houston, was founded by Jack Grayson, a visionary leader in the quality movement in the United States and a key player in the development of the Malcolm Baldrige Quality Award.

With the assistance of APQC consultants, the committee identified an approach that addressed the cost issue and covered all VA hospitals. The basic strategy in the approach selected was to begin with hired external consultants who would provide all consulting and training and then gradually phase in internal trainers and consultants to replace them. The strategy is summarized as follows:

1. Phase-in of implementation throughout the 172 VA hospitals over four years.

2. Development of a rollout model to include
   a. An implementation team, including a physician member, to work with each hospital
   b. Modification and utilization of private sector consulting and training materials
   c. Development of internal capabilities, to reduce reliance on external training and consulting
3. Establishment of a full-time executive assistant (coordinator) for TQI at each hospital
4. Establishment of a central focal point to coordinate all training activity.

Phase In Implementation Over Four Years

VHA leaders eventually settled on a systemwide rollout to consist of four overlapping phases over four to five years. Figure 6.1 shows the planned rollout.

This approach was selected for three reasons. First was the cost issue noted above. Frequently, when a government organization is

Figure 6.1. Original TQI Implementation Plan.

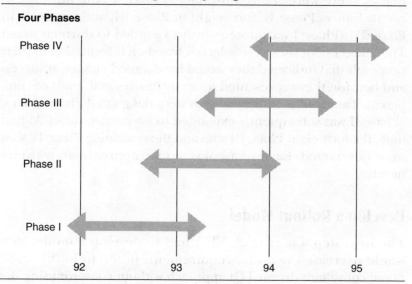

Four Phases

Phase IV

Phase III

Phase II

Phase I

92   93   94   95

faced with a costly process, it lengthens the time frame, thereby spending less money in a given fiscal year. Second, and equally important as the cost savings, was the advantage of gaining experience in a small number of hospitals before expanding the effort to other sites. Third, the phased-in approach allowed the development of a VHA-specific model by using input from the first hospitals to improve the TQI processes and training materials and to train VHA trainers and consultants. For this reason, hospitals in the first phase were called "pilot sites."

One of the first tasks was to determine which hospitals would go first. Concurrent with the formalized search for consultants, a second RFP was sent to all VA hospitals, asking for volunteers for the first phase. The RFP did not specify requirements; rather, it requested that hospitals describe their readiness to undertake TQI based on past activities and their willingness to provide funds to support their own TQI effort. The groundswell of interest surprised even VHA planners. More than one hundred hospitals applied. An ad hoc group composed of VHA staff, Federal Quality Institute staff, external consultants, and other federal quality leaders reviewed and ranked the applications and designated approximately one-third of the hospitals to be included in the first two phases.

The four-phase approach consisted of a geometric progression; that is, there were twelve hospitals in Phase I (the pilot sites), twenty-four in Phase II, forty-eight in Phase III, and ninety-six in Phase IV. (Phase I was subsequently expanded to thirteen sites.) The Phase I pilot sites were selected based on information in their proposals that indicated they would have a good chance at success and because they represented a variety of sizes and levels of complexity. Twenty-four additional sites were designated Phase II sites. (Phase II was subsequently expanded to twenty-five sites.) At that time, the forty-eight Phase III sites and the remaining Phase IV sites were not named. Each phase was to take approximately twelve months.

Develop a Rollout Model

The next step was crucial. VHA had to develop a model that would decrease the dollar requirements inherent in the traditional consultant-driven TQI approach without compromising the quality of implementation across the system. VHA was committed to moving from external to internal capability as quickly as possible. The model developed included three significant components: (1) the creation of "TQI teams" for each VA hospital, (2) conducting consultation and training events simultaneously, and (3) the development of internal capability.

Four-Member TQI Teams

Each hospital was assigned a special team to guide its introduction to TQI and its early experience with it. Each team consisted of a paid external consultant; a VHA trainer, who was simultaneously being trained to become a "master trainer"; a physician consultant from within VHA; and a member of the hospital staff, designated as the executive assistant for TQI. Each team member had specific roles and responsibilities.

The External Consultant

In the first two phases, all of the consultants were affiliated with APQC. The individual consultants were chosen by APQC for their experience in TQI implementation and, as much as possible, for their health care experience. They were to work closely with the leadership at the local site, especially with the executive assistants for TQI. Since TQI represented a relatively new management paradigm in most of the hospitals, the consultants spent a great deal of time introducing the concepts and working on the beginning steps. Because VA hospitals vary widely in size and complexity, consultants were expected to first become oriented to the hospital and its staff and then assist and advise them as they began implementing TQI. In those hospitals where TQI activities were already under way, the consultant was to provide a fresh external review to assist in assessing current strengths, gaps in knowledge and experience, and opportunities for improvement. They became involved in strategic quality planning and in launching process action teams and department-level quality deployment teams. They reported to the hospital management regularly about the progress of the TQI efforts. The consultants, with their extensive background in TQI, were the most knowledgeable members of the implementation teams and were seen as leaders.

The Physician Consultant

The private consultants had found in their previous experience that it was important to include clinicians in TQI efforts. They had learned that when doctors are confronted with new information or changed paradigms, they tend to relate better with other doctors than with management gurus. Their approach at non-VHA health care sites had been to bring in a physician who understood and embraced total quality to speak with the local physicians. APQC had one physician on their payroll who performed this function. Because of the large scope of the planned rollout and the inevitable fiscal constraints, VHA decided to develop its own group of physicians by enlisting volunteers from throughout the VHA health care system. Since the initial pilot sites were all starting their efforts together, VHA selected a total of twenty physicians. To the extent possible, the physicians selected were either already knowledgeable in total quality principles or at least were conversant with the quality improvement tools being introduced to hospital quality assurance functions under Galen Barbour's stewardship. The physician consultants were assembled early on in St. Louis for training.

One physician consultant was assigned to each VA hospital and traveled with the team to the site. Initially the physician consultant was scheduled to attend only the first meeting, but as implementation began, the role was expanded to include four or five visits. Early experiences taught that a single visit to a hospital by a physician consultant does not result in significant buy-in by the clinical staff. Therefore, the physician consultants looked for local physicians who showed the potential to become champions for total quality, and they spent the necessary time encouraging them to take a leading role. Drs. Galen Barbour, Frank Citro, and Robert Frymier took an early lead in developing the physician consultant program and in creating support structures, such as a telephone network, that were needed to ensure an effective cadre of physician champions.

The Master Trainers

VHA had an existing educational infrastructure that consisted of seven regional medical education centers (RMECs) and one continuing education center (CEC), which was devoted to centralized training efforts. The personnel at these centers included highly skilled educators, many with master's degrees or doctorates in education and clinical areas and all with experience in training VHA staff. The RMEC system had used and refined train-the-trainer approaches for certain courses, and thus it was already adept at developing the trainers and materials required for a "cascade" approach to training. Thus, when the TQI planning committee computed what it would cost to hire external trainers, they quickly came to the conclusion that it was much more cost-effective to train VHA personnel in the RMEC system. These VHA staff members would become the master trainers who would train the executive assistants for TQI and other hospital staff as needed to meet the ongoing demands of the implementation effort. A council of VHA educators made up of senior managers from the individual RMECs developed a plan that called for twenty-three of their staff to be trained as master trainers; these master trainers were then assigned to teams responsible for the pilot sites.

The master trainer candidates worked with the consultants to pilot-test the training materials before they were used at VA hospitals. The consultants trained them on the materials and later certified them after they demonstrated expert training skills. At Phase I pilot sites, they "shadowed" the consultants and began to coteach courses once they had completed the formal classroom training. In the second phase, the certified master trainers assumed responsibility for all of the training in the hospitals, under the observation of the hired consultants.

As the master trainers gained experience, they began to identify needed improvements in the original consultant-provided training materials. Their knowledge of the VHA health care system and of train-the-trainer techniques was used to develop a set of training materials with VHA-specific content. To this end, they spent much of their time in the pilot phase evaluating the materials, contributing additional VHA-specific content, developing appropriate formats, and field-testing the materials. They also identified additional content areas and support materials that needed to be developed. Also, an implementation guide, consisting of a notebook addressing each component of the rollout model, was developed by the consultants based on early feedback. This valuable guide provided essential information to staff involved in subsequent phases of the TQI implementation.

The Executive Assistant for TQI

The implementation plan called for an executive assistant for TQI position at each hospital. The role was to be multifaceted, with a primary focus on being an expert resource person and a facilitator. As the title suggests, the executive assistants for TQI were expected to take a leadership role in oversight, coordination, and training within the hospital. They acted as facilitators for leadership, the quality leadership team (QLT), and process action teams, and they served as the liaison between the process action teams and the quality leadership team. The consultants and VHA leadership recommended that the position be full-time. All VA hospitals had a "quality manager" responsible for traditional quality assurance functions; at the time, the executive assistant for TQI was seen as an additional role with unique responsibilities (discussed in greater detail below).

Simultaneous Consultation and Training

After the pilot phase, the external consultants modified the training manuals and gave them to VHA, with copying rights. When the potential cost was multiplied by the number of people to be trained, it was evident that VHA needed the right to print and distribute the manuals. Having such control over the training materials was important, because to purchase the materials from private sources would have cost from $25 to $150 per manual. Even when copyright questions were not an issue and trainers could legally copy manuals, local facilities did not always have the ability to copy large volumes in an efficient or professional manner. This arrangement also allowed VHA to update and revise the manuals over time.

Internal Capability

The implementation plan called for a significant decrease over time in VHA's reliance on private consulting support, with a commensurate increase in its reliance on VHA staff. The basic plan called for the following schedule of external consulting days at each hospital:

Days per Site	*Projected Costs*
Phase I: 96 days	$5.1 million
Phase II: 48 days	$2.7 million
Phase III: 24 days	$2.1 million
Phase IV: 12 days	$1.3 million

The decreasing costs reflect the decreasing reliance on paid consultants and an increasing reliance on in-house trainers and consultants. Figure 6.2 illustrates the relationship between VHA's reliance on external consultants and its in-house staff.

Develop an Internal TQI Expert

Developing an expert—an executive assistant for TQI—at each hospital was a linchpin of VHA's basic strategy. Selection of the individual was left to the discretion of the hospital director, as was the determination of whether the position would be full-time. In Phase I, little guidance was available on selecting an executive assistant for TQI, although most of those selected were good communicators, respected by their peers, and enthusiastic about TQI. Many were recruited from the ranks of quality managers at the hospitals.

Early planners of VHA's total quality journey recognized that developing the executive assistant for TQI position was critical to a successful outcome. They would be the internal resource persons and facilitators; in short, they would become the internal implementation consultant. Therefore, the external consultants at each hospital were to work extensively with the executive assistants for TQI and tutor them in the TQI process and the consultation skills they would need. In subsequent phases, new executive assistants for TQI would be offered the opportunity to visit an experienced hospital to "partner" with their counterpart. The experienced executive assistants for TQI could then assist in training their less experienced colleagues. This process also permitted a reduction in the number of external consulting days at future TQI sites. VHA was acutely aware of the importance of having skilled, dedicated workers in these positions; every step of the local TQI plan would hinge on having a strong and effective executive assistant for TQI in place.

**Figure 6.2. Phase-In Reliance on
VA Training Staff (FY 1991–1995).**

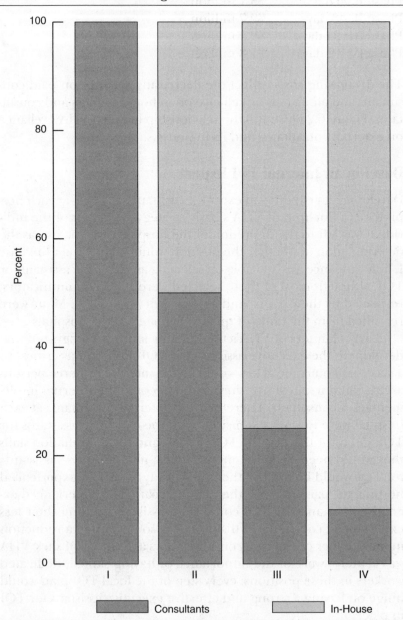

The specific plans for TQI implementation at each hospital—although locally developed—would follow similar steps across the system. Variety in programs and settings among different VA hospitals required flexibility in their approach to implementation. The diversity of VHA was especially apparent from the range of facilities appearing on the list of TQI pilot sites. There were twelve hospitals and one independent outpatient clinic (Columbus, OH), representing facilities both large and small, rural and urban, and complex and simple.

Albany, NY	Albuquerque, NM	Brooklyn, NY
Big Spring, TX	Columbus, OH	Danville, IL
Indianapolis, IN	Lexington, KY	Loma Linda, CA
New York, NY	Oklahoma City, OK	Prescott, AZ
Tuscaloosa, AL		

On the other hand, Phase II sites were selected predominantly by their readiness and willingness to embrace TQI, creating somewhat of a geographic imbalance:

Bay Pines, FL	Charleston, SC	Chicago, IL (West Side)
Cleveland, OH	Dallas, TX	Dayton, OH
Fresno, CA	Grand Junction, CO	Jackson, MS
Las Vegas, NV	Long Beach, CA	Memphis, TN
Minneapolis, MN	Phoenix, AZ	Portland, OR
Reno, NV	San Antonio, TX	San Diego, CA
Spokane, WA	St. Louis, MO	Temple, TX
Togus, ME	Tucson, AZ	Walla Walla, WA
White City, OR		

Twelve of the Phase II sites (48 percent) were located in VHA's western region. This was no accident; rather, it reflected the early commitment to TQI principles made by that region's leadership and the involvement of several clinical leaders. Planners used the pilot sites' experiences to develop a set of practices and principles that would be employed at succeeding sites: establishing a governing body, creating mission and vision statements, conducting quality assessments, providing training, and launching performance improvement teams.

A two-day initial visit gave key staff an opportunity to meet the consulting team. These visits would include an introductory interview with senior management, the director, the chief of staff, and the associate director, along with a series of interviews with mid-level managers (service chiefs) and other key staff to get their views on TQI philosophy, important issues facing the facility, and existing TQI activities. At the end of the two-day visit, an exit meeting with senior management would summarize the information and set dates for the next steps in the TQI implementation.

The plan called for each facility to establish a TQI governing body, such as a quality leadership team (QLT), normally made up of senior and mid-level management. These individuals were responsible for monitoring and providing oversight of TQI activities in general; managing the assessment process; developing mission, vision, and values; creating the strategic quality plan, which would include the TQI training plan; and launching the cultural improvement and process improvement teams.

The plan also called for an "envisioning workshop," a one- to one-and-a-half-day session designed to help the leadership team define the facility's organizational mission (the purpose of the organization), vision (what the facility would be in the future), and values (the principles that would guide the facility). These were to be shared and endorsed by all employees. Also, as part of the workshop the leadership team would identify and prioritize key processes in preparation for the organizational assessment.

The objective of the assessment was to

- Examine and analyze policies, practices, and systems
- Establish a quality baseline using the seven elements of the Malcolm Baldrige National Quality Award (a world-class standard)
- Develop a quality improvement plan

It would be conducted by a mix of facility staff under the guidance of the external consultant, and it would end with a report to the QLT. The leadership team would then use the data and information collected to set priorities and to help them make decisions in the strategic quality planning session.

The next step in the implementation process was the development of the strategic quality plan by the leadership team, in a two-day session facilitated by the consultants, following completion of the assessment. This written plan would outline priorities for cross-functional process improvement, cultural improvement, and service-level TQI implementation. It would also include a preliminary time line for launching and training teams, using the process performance data and external customer feedback to establish priorities.

Unfortunately, plans frequently don't go as anticipated— especially in a large, diverse organization like VHA. Flexibility was key to building strong working relationships between consultants, VHA master trainers, and hospital staff. The initial Phase I hospitals were selected early in the spring of 1991, but delays prevented implementation until August 1991. Since the initial visits were scheduled between August and November 1991, the twelve-week time frame for several fell into the Thanksgiving and Christmas holidays, making it difficult for the assessment teams to complete their work before the end of January 1992. The Phase I plenary session, which was supposed to have occurred before start-up, was rescheduled to February 1992. The emphasis for this meeting thus changed from planning for implementation to redesign of the implementation for the remainder of Phase I and the start-up of Phase II. The plenary session for Phase II facilities was held in April 1992, ahead of the scheduled start-up in July.

At the end of each phase of implementation, the consulting teams were to transition out of the facilities after completing their first-year TQI implementation. Part of the transition process involved a meeting in which the consulting team and the leadership team worked together to evaluate their progress and establish their TQI plans for the subsequent year. The diversity in the individual hospitals and the variation in the timing of their implementation scheduling underscored the need for some form of coordinating activity.

Coordinate All VHA TQI Training

As the plan for TQI implementation was being developed, a structure was also developed to direct, implement, and support all of the TQI activities. The Office of Resource Management remained the "owner" of the TQI process. The project was headed by John Fears, and he designated individuals within his office to continue strategic planning as well as to monitor the day-to-day operations of the TQI effort. The contract with the external consultants was written and administered by that office, which was also responsible for decisions about all issues that arose at the field sites.

The Office of Resource Management requested that the Office of Academic Affairs (which managed the RMECs) designate one of its staff to be responsible for coordinating and supporting all TQI training. Thus the Center for TQI Education was established at the St. Louis continuing education center. The responsibilities of the TQI training center included

- Coordinating TQI training assignments
- Monitoring TQI training
- Preparing reports required for TQI training
- Administering the TQI training budget
- Organizing travel for all TQI training activities
- Purchasing TQI materials
- Developing and monitoring additional contracts
- Developing and maintaining communications links
- Addressing the ongoing education needs of TQI participants

The training center began with a staff of four individuals to support the multiple activities required. Each of the seven RMECs designated three persons from their current staff, or they hired additional personnel, to become master trainers. One of the three at each RMEC served as team leader. A program assistant was assigned at each RMEC for the administrative support needed by the TQI team.

The TQI training center was important to achieving VHA's goal of establishing a common approach to TQI, in terms of basic principles and tools that would facilitate exchange of information, personnel, and experiences between hospitals. Staff with experience at one hospital could move to another and proceed with minimal reorientation. The training center was able to maintain a uniform training package and to ensure that trainers delivered the materials consistently. It established a systematic communication flow that enabled trainers to bring problems to the surface quickly and get solutions that were rapidly disseminated to all other trainers. It was also able to establish regular communications with the executive assistants for TQI, through monthly conference calls, and to give them a forum for addressing complaints and problems. In essence, the training center became the hub around which the wheels of VHA's TQI effort revolved.

This, in short, was VHA's plan for implementing a new way of doing business: roll out in phases, jump start with paid consultants, develop in-house capability as rapidly as possible, and coordinate the massive amount of training needed through a central training center. The following chapters describe the events that actually occurred when this plan was implemented.

Part Three

From Theory
to Practice

Linking Physicians to the Process

Steven R. Orwig

Previous chapters have addressed the evolution of total quality improvement (TQI), from its roots in manufacturing to its adaptation by service industries and then to its application in health care in the late 1980s. This chapter discusses one of the implications of this last shift: the necessity of dealing with clinicians. In this chapter, the term *clinician* refers to physicians, registered nurses, physician assistants, nurse practitioners, pharmacists, psychologists, social workers, dietitians, and all the many others who are directly involved in delivering patient care. Since there are some unique and especially significant issues associated with physicians, I will make it clear when I am dealing specifically with them.

Clinicians and TQI

Clinical staff present special opportunities and obstacles, unique to the hospital setting, in implementing TQI efforts. On the one hand, clinicians have a customer (patient) focus, experience with cross-functional teams, and a data-driven approach to their work, attributes that favor acceptance of TQI. On the other hand, clinicians exhibit paternalism, have a lack of appreciation for the importance of *internal* customers, tend to be skeptical about the efficacy of TQI efforts, and have many competing responsibilities and thus a lack of time. These characteristics hinder acceptance of

TQI. Further, one result of the division of hospitals into clinical and administrative functions (a situation for which there is no exact parallel in most other working environments) is that clinicians are often tempted to see any initiative that comes from "the front office" as being outside their primary sphere of interest and certainly secondary to their role of taking care of patients.

In the Veterans Health Administration (VHA)—and probably in other health care organizations as well—two common but inaccurate associations made by clinicians have reinforced their tendency to reject TQI. First, many clinicians equate TQI with the quality assurance (QA) measures of the past. Many have had negative experiences with the audits, reviews, reports, and plans mandated by QA efforts (especially those prior to 1991). Although one can hardly argue with the goal of ensuring quality, few clinicians are convinced that the types of QA activities they have traditionally participated in really have a beneficial effect on patient care. Physicians, in particular, view QA activities as a search for "bad apples"— and they have often been the targets of such searches. Further, most physicians do not feel that the ministrations of the QA office actually accomplish much of anything in the way of improving medical outcomes. Since many clinicians see TQI as an extension or outgrowth of QA, these negative connotations are part of the mental picture they have constructed of TQI. Some consultants have attempted to avoid this by downplaying the things TQI and QA have in common and stressing how they differ. This resulted in presentations where the features of the old, shortsighted, ineffective, punitive QA methods were contrasted with the new, insightful, efficacious, scientific principles of TQI. Such simplistic expositions probably did more to disparage QA (and the people who carried it out) than they did to elevate TQI, but it is not hard to see why such an approach might have seemed necessary.

Second, many clinicians associate TQI with the Joint Commission on Accreditation of Healthcare Organizations (JCAHO). TQI implementation in VHA coincided not only with JCAHO's growing emphasis on quality improvement but also with VHA's endeavors to improve its relationship with the Joint Commission by (among other things) establishing JCAHO training sessions for hospital directors, physician and nursing leaders, and QA staff. Further, in many hospitals, the same staff members were responsible for QA activities, JCAHO compliance, and TQI efforts, so these came to be seen as inextricably linked. As with QA, the stated mission of the JCAHO—"to improve the quality of care provided to the public"—is certainly one that clinicians should embrace, but (also like QA) many clinicians see JCAHO as some citizens see government: a well-intentioned enterprise gone out of control. They associate JCAHO with time-consuming efforts to generate structures, policies, and documentation that seem to add no value beyond helping to satisfy slippery, legalistic interpretations of ambiguous standards. Understandably, these images have done nothing to endear TQI to clinical staff.

Of course, not all clinicians disapprove of QA departments or JCAHO requirements, and not all of those who do disapprove of them connect TQI with them. But for those who do, TQI has had two strikes against it from the outset.

Patients as Customers

Many elements of TQI come naturally to clinicians, but some others seem irrelevant or inconsistent. This tension can be demonstrated in a number of different areas. For example, TQI organizations must be "customer-oriented," putting the customer in a position of paramount importance—and that is just how clinicians view patients. But even though clinicians recognize that patients are ultimately the reason for their professional existence, our formal education generally has not prepared us to assess and respond to the nontechnical, subjective aspects of patient care that often contribute most to a patient's sense of satisfaction. Physicians, especially, are trained to acquire information from patients and evaluate their response to treatment. We readily recognize patients' needs for competent, accessible, comprehensive care, but many of us are less attuned to their wishes for privacy, physical comfort, emotional support, and involvement in decision making. Surveys and focus groups show that patients often feel these factors are inadequately addressed by doctors. So, even though clinicians want to do what is best for patients (that is, our customers), our idea of what is best does not always agree with the patients' ideas. (This conflict in how quality of care is defined is discussed further under Lesson 4, below.)

No less important is the fact that the term *customer* presents a semantic problem. In the teaching of TQI, the customer occupies a lofty place indeed. The customer's response is the barometer of any organizational activity's success. However, many (perhaps most) clinicians are put off the first time they hear patients referred to as customers or clients, because they find these terms demeaning and depersonalizing. For many, *customer* has mercantile connotations that are too crass to reconcile with their idea of the proper clinician-patient relationship. John Farrar, M.D., acting chief medical director for VHA after James Holsinger's departure, spoke for many physicians when he said he believes that every time we call a patient a customer, an angel dies.

To complicate matters even further, many clinicians have trouble with the notion of *internal* customers. For example, physicians tend to view nurses, pharmacists, laboratory staff, and other clinicians only as suppliers or processors in the TQI model rather than as customers, which they actually are in many circumstances.

Cross-Functional Teams, Data, and Processes

TQI emphasizes the use of cross-functional teams, and most clinicians have experience working on such teams. Operating rooms, clinics, and inpatient wards are a few examples of areas where several different disciplines work together. However, these are often *multi*disciplinary groups, where each person's contribution is essentially independent of and parallel to what the others do, as opposed to *inter*disciplinary teams, where the various participants communicate and cooperate interdependently. To physicians used to a "captain-of-the-ship" model, interdependence may seem like an inefficient indulgence. One chief of staff expressed a lack of enthusiasm for TQI precisely because of this emphasis on teams. He feared that under this new philosophy, no decision would be made without assembling a team to analyze the implications, and he envisioned that this would paralyze all decision making. This concern, shared by many hospital administrators, is often accompanied by concern that without clear-cut lines of responsibility among hospital staff, personal accountability will be lost and most workers will feel that process improvement is "not my job."

Some physicians are leery of teams for a few other reasons as well. Participating in teams takes much more time than simply making a decision and moving on. Diffusing decision making within the clinical setting directly affects physicians' autonomy. In the world of private practice, time is money; time spent on teamwork might represent lost income. This situation does not pertain in VHA, where physicians are salaried employees of the system. But the time requirement is still of concern to VHA physicians, who are nevertheless extremely busy.

TQI demands that changes be data-driven, and clinicians are accustomed to measuring and responding to objective data. Yet, clinicians (especially physicians) are often skeptical that TQI can be effectively transported from manufacturing settings to health care, doubting the validity of much of the data generated in support of TQI teams. Part of this questioning attitude is based in clinicians' not wanting to give up familiar methods of making decisions, including the "wise man" approach. There is not a general fear of measurement, since clinicians are certainly used to looking at data. But the data most clinicians work with pertains to individual patients, while process improvement requires a more epidemiologic approach. To engage in TQI, clinicians must be prepared to analyze data from groups of patients and cohorts of people with similar demographics. This is not an area in which most physicians are trained.

At a more fundamental level, clinicians (like most people) do not readily embrace "process thinking." For example, when faced with a patient with a cough and fever, one clinician (typically a physician) will collect and evaluate the pertinent data, make a diagnosis, and prescribe treatment. Others are then responsible for seeing that the orders are delivered to the appropriate place, that the prescribed drug is accurately dispensed and correctly administered, that requested monitoring is initiated, and that these actions are appropriately documented. Such a division of labor may be natural and efficient, but it tends to obscure the fact that these tasks are all part of a single process. Unless the entire process fits together smoothly, patient care will suffer. Such processes abound in health care, and they work optimally only if all of those involved—physicians, other clinicians, and nonclinical personnel—understand how each contribution fits into the whole.

Finally, health care workers are not exempt from the barriers to TQI that are encountered in any other setting. The universal complaints of too little time and too many competing responsibilities provoke health care's version of the fundamental TQI lament: "We wouldn't have so many patient complaints if we didn't have to attend all these meetings."

For all of the preceding reasons and more, many clinicians approach TQI with skepticism. This fact has important implications for how a health care organization will begin incorporating TQI principles, particularly how it will address the fundamental questions of physician involvement: when and how.

Organizational Approaches to Clinician Involvement

Lesson 6 of Berwick, Godfrey, and Roessner's Ten Key Lessons for Quality Improvement (1990) says "Involving Doctors Is Difficult"; a few of the reasons for this have been described above. If this is true, then their Lesson 8, "Nonclinical Processes Draw Early Attention," must follow as a corollary. Some organizations deal with physician resistance to TQI by looking only at administrative processes in the beginning. Choosing to avoid clinical issues in the early stages is a plausible strategy. It is legitimate to ask whether it is really necessary to involve physicians early in the implementation effort. Perhaps by avoiding the complications of physician participation in the initial learning phase, the organization can more easily acquire experience, achieve some initial successes, and develop a cadre of team leaders and facilitators. In this way, it might improve its chances of successfully involving physicians at a later point.

In spite of the allure of this argument, there are risks. First, lessons learned in teams that do not include physicians may not easily extend to teams that do. Second, this approach tends to reinforce the popular misconception that TQI works with administrative processes but not with clinical ones. Third, not involving physicians from the beginning may attach an "outsider" status to them that will be difficult to alter later. And finally, many processes identified as nonclinical really do affect clinicians. When we ignore or suppress that connection, we lessen the likelihood of sustaining improvement; plus we make it more difficult to counter the clinical-administrative division that exists in most health care settings.

Because of these concerns, many deem it wiser to involve physicians from the beginning, in spite of the difficulties. This was the approach taken by VHA, both at the national level and at most of its hospitals.

The VHA Approach to Clinician Involvement

Given that clinicians (and especially physicians) require special consideration, organizers of VHA's TQI effort decided early on to recruit physician consultants to visit each implementation site. The rationale was clear: skeptical clinicians are more readily persuaded by "one of their own." Someone whose first loyalty is patient care makes a more credible advocate for the utility and efficacy of clinical TQI applications.

For the thirteen Phase I pilot sites, organizers in the headquarters Office of Quality Management and the St. Louis continuing education center (CEC) identified VHA physicians and dentists with previous interest, experience, and enthusiasm for quality improvement. Seven of the sixteen individuals—two of them dentists—selected to serve as internal (VHA) physician consultants to the Phase I hospitals came from the Hines VA hospital in Chicago, the site of John Fears's early success. The other Phase I consultants were mostly chiefs of staff from hospitals that were already beginning to endorse the concepts of continuous improvement; a few were from VHA headquarters or RMEC sites. As described in Chapter 6, these physician consultants were individually assigned to a Phase I hospital and visited it with an external consultant and a master trainer during the initial portion of the site's introduction and assessment activities. VHA considered the "core four" (the external consultant, the physician consultant, the master trainer, and the facility's executive assistant for TQI) to be the heart of the implementation team. Some of the physician consultants made additional trips to their assigned facility if requested by the director and if funding permitted. On these trips they were often asked to meet with facility physicians singly or in groups to discuss the role of physicians in the TQI process.

These physician consultants also initiated a monthly conference call among themselves to discuss issues and problems at their sites. In the beginning these calls were arranged and hosted by

Lynn Ward at the St. Louis CEC; but in midsummer 1992 the responsibility for the physician consultant program was shifted to the Office of Quality Management, and the conference call became the responsibility of Frank Citro, M.D.

During the monthly calls, several different topics were discussed concerning the general role of physician consultants in the various hospitals. At almost every site, the role of the physician consultant seemed somewhat ambiguous; most of the physician consultants agreed, however, that in those facilities with clear and obvious endorsement and involvement by top management (the triad of hospital director, associate director, and chief of staff) the process ran more smoothly. This was a lesson learned and relearned over and over by the various facilities: top management involvement is crucial.

The Phase I physician consultants made some critical observations regarding the assessment process, the outside consultants, and the role of future physician consultants. They found several shortcomings in the assessment methodology, centering around, as one physician put it, "the lack of any connection between the assessment process and what the hospital should be doing—patient care." In addition to this lack of clinical emphasis, they noted that the assessments were far too broad and sweeping in their focus and that participants were not given the information or training they needed to make anything specific from the broad generalizations. The physician consultants noted that the facilities were often left with very broad areas for improvement. Similarly, the master trainers later noted that the assessment topics chosen for the first few teams at each facility were far too encompassing (a "solve-world-hunger" type of charter). Lastly, the physician consultants were not impressed with the use of Baldrige-type structures in the assessment process; their impression was that most of the hospitals were not ready for that degree of sophistication in the assessment process. This concern led directly to one of their most cogent recommendations—that VHA develop a health care–specific assessment tool, preferably possessing some relevance to VHA as a whole as well, for its primary assessment tool rather than relying on a tool developed for industry. (The development of this tool is discussed in Chapter Ten.)

In their monthly conference calls, the physician consultants discussed the fact that the outside consultants did not have any significant hospital background and seemed to be relying on them for guidance in specifics about health care; it had not been at all clear to most of the physician consultants that this would be the case. This was not the only example of poor communication between the members of the "core four." In fact, the physician consultants noted on several occasions that the concept of the "core four" team simply did not work—training materials were not presented at the facilities beforehand; the physician consultants were not told what, if any, part of the presentation to the steering committee could be given by them; and there was no planning for the committee meetings on the part of the other team members (everyone generally met in the lobby of the hotel on the first morning as they were on their way to meet with the steering committee). Here, as well, the physician consultants had good concrete suggestions about improving the process and their role: they recommended that the "core four" begin operating as a team, with all its members receiving materials to review ahead of meeting times and by meeting together, if only by telephone, prior to arriving at the steering committee meetings. They also strongly urged that the role of the physician consultant be strengthened in Phase II rather than diminished. They clearly felt that their presence had been of some value to the hospitals, although they also pointed out some flaws in logistics that made their participation more difficult. For example, more attention needed to be paid to their schedules when planning the steering committee meetings—the dates had been set with everyone else before checking with them, and some had missed an opportunity to attend because of conflicts. They all agreed that they should have more material to present to the local physicians—material such as articles about the importance of physician involvement in TQI and stories about successful implementations of TQI in other health care settings, especially other VA hospitals.

Many of the changes to the physician consultant component of Phase II were suggested by the physician consultants themselves. Often these suggestions were first made in the conference calls; they were formally incorporated into the training materials for Phase II at a plenary session in Reno, Nevada, in February 1992. Points stressed by the physician consultants at that meeting included the importance of their early involvement, their usefulness in helping their local facility get its own physicians involved, and their importance in overseeing the clinical aspects of the program. Most of the Phase I physician consultants again served as consultants for some of the twenty-five Phase II facilities.

On the basis of the experience of the Phase I physician consultants, active recruiting of additional consultants for Phase II was undertaken to provide a large enough pool of talent to allow individual consultants to spend more time at each facility. Prospective candidates were judged on their knowledge of and experience with the quality improvement process, the degree of credibility they would carry into a site, and their personal endorsement of the cardinal features of the quality improvement process: employee involvement, teamwork, and data-driven decisions. Lastly, the new consultants were chosen for their ability to inspire and lead other physicians to also become enthused and involved. They and their supervisors were made aware that a five- to seven-day minimum commitment away from their primary work site would be required.

Training for these physician consultants consisted primarily of a two-day meeting in St. Louis on June 8–10, 1992, shortly before the kickoff of Phase II. The objectives of this training session were to ensure that the participants understood the philosophy of TQI as it pertains to process and outcome measures in health care; how this philosophy relates to the interactions between TQI, traditional QA, and JCAHO requirements; and how to use this knowledge to assess the effectiveness of the major processes in a health care institution. Consultants from the American Productivity and Quality Center (APQC) outlined their approach to the rollout, and the physician consultants then discussed their responsibilities, the obstacles they might encounter, and some of the resources available to help them overcome those barriers. Since physician involvement was seen to be such a critical factor for a fully successful TQI effort, the consultants' first and foremost responsibility was to help maximize physician "buy-in."

Most of the discussion concerned anticipating the different kinds of resistance that might be encountered and then developing strategies for dealing with it. Much time was spent in planning for the collection and circulation of "success stories," cases where TQI principles had been applied with favorable results. The group established fairly strict criteria for the type of success story that would be most effective. First, they insisted that only examples from health care settings be used. Management consultants gushed with illustrations from auto manufacturers, hotel chains, fast-food restaurants, and clothing retailers, but the participants agreed that these did little to persuade hospital staff that the same approaches would work in health care. Second, they wanted examples of improvements in *clinical* processes. Again, skeptical clinicians would not be greatly impressed by increased efficiency in the laundry service or improved reagent acquisitions in the laboratory. Clinicians *are* impressed by decreased infection or mortality rates, improved control of hypertension or pain, and delayed progression of renal dysfunction or retinopathy. Somewhere between these extremes were examples of improvements that straddle the clinical-administrative boundary, such as increased medical record availability in the clinic, decreased operating room turnaround times, and quicker prescription fills by the outpatient pharmacy; still, participants had mixed responses regarding how valuable these examples would prove in demonstrating to a clinician that TQI could improve patient care.

To further increase the usefulness and accessibility of success stories, physician consultants at the Phase II training session created a success-story template, consisting of a clear title for the story; a brief history of the problem; a short description of how the problem was addressed, including the composition of any team initiated to solve it; the intervention made; and the pre- and postintervention data, followed by a report of the outcome of the intervention and a short moral to be learned from the story. The template was used for the collection and reporting of these stories, which were placed in a central database. Consultants were encouraged to look for examples of success stories in their travels and submit them to the database regularly.

It is important not to overlook some of the limitations of success stories. Successful process improvement efforts can suggest possible areas for improvement, demonstrate that a shared problem is fixable, point out unsuspected obstacles, and show one way to deal with a particular problem. But teams that try to "plug in" another hospital's solutions are typically disappointed. The problem they face could be subtly but critically different from the one described in the success story. They might neglect subtle but critical elements of the successful intervention, elements that even the successful group may not have appreciated. Regardless, the journey is often more important than the destination. Although teams may complain that they are reinventing the wheel, the insight and rapport gained by completely and thoroughly analyzing the process yields great rewards. Interestingly, more than one consultant observed that, in many cases, "failure stories" were more instructive for demonstrating TQI principles than success stories (though they may not be the best way to prove the potential benefits of TQI).

As stated above, the primary role of the physician consultants at Phase I and II facilities was to increase acceptance and participation by the medical staff. Secondary roles were to facilitate buy-in from other clinicians and to provide the clinical perspective for nonclinician participants. After the training session in St. Louis, each Phase II hospital was again assigned a "core four" composed of an APQC consultant, who served as the TQI content and process expert; a RMEC master trainer, who assisted in training needs; an executive assistant for TQI; and a physician consultant. The plan called for the physician to make four visits, usually over a period of four to eight months, from the initial rollout to the end of the facility assessment and strategic planning session, and to be involved in a variety of implementation functions at the facility.

Physician consultants used various approaches to encourage clinician involvement, among them making presentations to the medical staff, meeting with individual physician leaders, and attending meetings of process action teams and quality leadership teams (QLTs). Their presentations typically covered the history and rationale of TQI and included success stories from the consultant's own facility or from the experience of other physician consultants. Probably more important than any specific content, however, was the physician's being present and describing positive experiences with TQI from a clinical point of view.

Between the time of the training and mid-February 1993, a period of eight months, the physician consultants visited twenty-three of the twenty-five Phase II sites (the others were not visited because of scheduling problems between the facility, the physician consultant, and the rest of the "core team"). Six of the facilities were visited for only two days, but all the others received four or more days of physician consultation time—one received nine days and three received ten days of consultation. In a survey conducted by the St. Louis CEC in July 1993, physician consultants and hospital directors were asked, independently, to rate their experiences. Seven of the hospital directors reported that their experience with their physician consultant was not positive; they found their consultant to be detached, uncommitted, unhelpful, or, at the very least, inexperienced. The majority of directors, including most of the seven with negative experiences, wanted to have an outside physician consultant and indicated that the benefit was greatest when the physician was experienced in TQI and could spend more than just a few days at the facility. They felt that the presence of a physician consultant added credibility to the implementation effort with their local clinical staff, but in the future they wanted to pick the consultant who would come to their facility.

Fourteen of the twenty-two physician consultants thought the experience had been helpful. Four believed that the time they had spent consulting had definitely not been useful, and the remaining four were uncertain of the value of their consultations. Those that felt they had been useful believed that their successes were in convincing the local physicians of the value of the TQI approach, sharing ideas and success stories, and bringing a clinical perspective to the proceedings. They recommended further training for themselves or subsequent physician consultants, with particular attention on working on a consulting team, having a clear definition of the physician consultant role, and obtaining some consulting experience and knowledge of past experience with TQI within VHA.

Predictably, reactions from physicians at the implementation sites varied. Brent James, M.D., of Intermountain Health Care suggested that about one-third of physicians "are current or potential [TQI] leaders," one-third "are relatively passive," and the remaining third "are difficult to convince and . . . will raise many objections" (Geehr & Pine, 1992, pp. 39–40.) Those proportions may actually be optimistic, but many consultants have described a similar division of responses.

Interviews with some of the master trainers uncovered some interesting relationships between the attributes of the facilities and those of the physician consultants. The greatest level of physician involvement and interest occurred in those sites where there was an obvious endorsement from top management, including the chief of staff, and acceptance by the informal leadership as well. When only the chief of staff was involved or where the top leadership's attendance was poor, physician involvement was correspondingly low. At White City Domiciliary, the commitment of the chief of staff, Mike Kelly, was obvious, and his expectations of the physician staff and the results of the TQI process were well known. Kelly was responsible for the site's rapid, just-in-time feedback on all team activity. As one physician explained, since the clinical staff could see what was happening, they knew what was important and their participation was correspondingly high. A physician-led team in the alcohol and drug treatment program at White City was able to reduce their cycle time for initial patient assessments and development of treatment plans from fourteen days to three days.

The Pittsburgh University Drive VA hospital experienced a lot of physician involvement, including from bedside caregivers. The quality coordinator at that site, Barbara Reichbaum, said, "Some of the greatest supporters at University Drive are the 'hands on' physicians—they clearly believe that interdisciplinary attention to the processes and technique of care will improve patient care and outcomes." In Pittsburgh, like many other sites where physician involvement was high, the key to success was the participation and leadership of two or three key informal physician leaders. Even in those facilities where physicians did become heavily involved, there was a tendency for them to gravitate toward serving on the QLT or in other leadership roles in the various teams. As they experienced the "Aha!" phenomenon of seeing process improvement affect patient outcomes, they often became more deeply involved team members.

Clinicians who did get involved took any of a number of different paths:

- Participating in QLTs
- Participating in assessments and strategic planning
- Participating in or leading process teams
- Consulting to process teams
- Assisting in implementing changes recommended by process teams

Most VA hospital QLTs included physicians and other clinicians besides the chief of staff. The Portland hospital QLT counted eight physicians among its nineteen members, and they reported good attendance and participation (that degree of physician representation on a QLT was unusual, however). Two to five physician members on a QLT was more typical of the Phase I and II hospitals' experience.

Clinicians were well represented during hospital assessments and strategic planning. The thirty-two employees of the Oklahoma City VA hospital who played active roles in their eight-week TQI assessments in 1991 included eight physicians and eleven other clinicians. All of these nineteen clinicians were intimately involved with collecting data, identifying problems, and prioritizing process improvement opportunities.

Interestingly, some physicians who were unenthusiastic about TQI *theory* latched onto the TQI *process* to bring about changes in areas of interest to them. For example, physicians at the Walla Walla VA hospital envisioned an ambitious restructuring of their inpatient and outpatient systems. They created a private practice–model team led by a physician and including representatives from nursing, medical administration, pharmacy, and others. This team developed a time line, visited a hospital with a similar system, planned staffing and space changes, identified barriers, designed work flow processes, and successfully switched to the new system, in spite of untimely staff losses and other distractions (including a JCAHO accreditation visit). Some of the physicians who were most actively involved in these impressive changes were skeptical of many parts of the TQI implementation effort.

Another example of a clinician-led process action team is the Albany VA hospital's hip-replacement team. Cochaired by an orthopedic surgeon and a physiatrist, this team began as a means of exploring cost-effectiveness issues even before the hospital officially launched its TQI implementation. Once the quality leadership team was formed, the hip-replacement team was reorganized and sanctioned as a TQI process improvement team. Using a clinical pathway approach, this group redesigned some of the processes for treating arthroplasty patients and achieved quantifiable improvements in patient satisfaction and cost-effectiveness of care.

Within two years of beginning their TQI journey, some VA

hospitals had launched more than two dozen teams. Virtually all included clinicians, and a great many had physician members, even those teams that dealt with such obviously nonclinical areas as parking or reward and recognition. Further, even teams that include clinicians frequently call in other clinicians to serve in an advisory or consultative capacity.

Finally, clinicians are often called on to assist in the implementation of recommendations made by process improvement teams. Care must be taken to ensure good communication and to generate broad ownership in any proposed modifications, so that important stakeholders do not feel ignored or perceive that the changes are arbitrary.

Lessons Learned

Comments from hospital-based physicians, physician consultants, and senior managers at several hospitals revealed that certain patterns of physician (and other clinician) involvement in and valuing of TQI had appeared. The major lessons learned in the Phase I and Phase II implementation efforts include the following:

1. *Physicians frequently respond differently from other clinicians.* In general, physicians seem to be less willing than other clinicians to accept the potential benefits of TQI. (But remember, all generalizations are false.) For some this is the result of cynicism or a lack of faith in anything that appears nonclinical, nonacademic, or otherwise foreign. For most, however, it merely reflects a healthy scientific skepticism that will respond to rational arguments and objective evidence. For clinicians, the important question regarding TQI is "Can this really improve patient care, or is it just going to take time away from seeing patients?" Or, more simply, "Does it work?" As described above in the Walla Walla example, often the ones who are most vocal in their skepticism will become the most active physician participants on process improvement teams. Several consultants noted that the physicians who do not say anything at all, positive or negative, in response to a TQI presentation generally prove to be the hardest to convince that TQI is worthwhile.

2. *Semantic issues are common and important.* As mentioned above, many clinicians are put off by the term *customer*. Many other words and phrases can impede meaningful communication because they have multiple meanings *(process, mission)*, are ambiguous *(culture)*, or have lost meaning through overuse *(paradigm, paradigm shift)*. As tends to happen with any structured activity, TQI has acquired its own technical language, which sometimes crosses the line between a customized lexicon for succinctly expressing complex thoughts and a lazy jargon that obscures meaning. We must always keep in mind that the message that is sent is not always the message that is received. An example of this occurred during one TQI steering committee meeting where a physician told the group, "I think we have a problem with clinic waiting times." The executive assistant for TQI replied, "This is not a 'problem'! It's an 'opportunity for improvement'!" The executive assistant was trying to avoid negative language and to emphasize, in the spirit of *kaizen*, that they were presented with a chance to make the system better. But the physician heard this response as an attempt to whitewash the difficulty and avoid facing it squarely.

3. *The need for measurement is underappreciated, and getting useful data is hard.* Clinicians are usually receptive to the idea that action will be based on objective measurements, but the effort required to design and obtain such measurements is almost always underestimated. Berwick, Godfrey, and Roessner (1990) pointed out that data for quality improvement abound in health care, but they also noted that hospital databases are often "not focused on the problems at hand" (p. 148). Establishing a valid and reliable measure of the performance of the process being studied is probably the step that is most often neglected. Teams commonly adopt an existing statistic and then discover a few months down the road that it does not provide the information they wanted. An example of this issue can be found in one of the first process improvement teams at the Oklahoma City VA hospital, which looked at waiting times in the hospital's walk-in clinic. The team found that they could easily get average disposition times (that is, the time from check-in to check-out) from the hospital computer. After several months of collecting and graphing these data, the team discovered (to its surprise) that this was not particularly meaningful

information, so they developed several other measures—number of patients awaiting complete treatment at 5:00 P.M., number of patients with a disposition time greater than four hours, and so on—which they found to be more useful and more reliable.

4.   *TQI in manufacturing is not the same as TQI in health care.* "Zero defects" is not an appropriate or helpful goal when dealing with biological systems. In manufacturing, quality is defined by the customer. In health care, there are aspects of quality that patients are not equipped to judge. While patients can certainly evaluate timeliness, courtesy, or the effectiveness of patient education, they are rarely in a position to appraise technical skills, fund of knowledge, or clinical judgment. For example, Dr. A sees Mr. X promptly, asks about his family, and thoroughly explains the medication he prescribes. However, he misdiagnoses Mr. X's problem, delaying effective treatment for six weeks. Dr. B makes Mr. Y wait an hour and a half past his scheduled appointment time, spends less than five minutes with him, and fails to answer all of Mr. Y's questions. He prescribes the correct treatment, and Mr. Y recovers quickly. Which patient is more likely to be satisfied with the quality of his care? (Reaching the correct diagnosis does not excuse unfriendly behavior.)

5.   *You won't convince everyone.* Not all clinicians will participate; identify the strategic few who will. All it takes is for them to see that TQI is effective in bringing about changes they feel are important. Do not underestimate what can be accomplished when only a few members of the physician staff are open and enthusiastic.

References

Berwick, D. M., Godfrey, A. B., & Roessner, J. (1990). *Curing health care: New strategies for quality improvement.* San Francisco: Jossey-Bass.

Geehr, E. C., & Pine, J. (1992). *Increasing physician involvement in quality improvement programs.* Tampa, FL: American College of Physician Executives.

Chapter Eight

Building a Foundation of Leadership

David K. Lee

At the time the Veterans Health Administration (VHA) was beginning its total quality improvement (TQI) implementation, most data surrounding successful TQI efforts were from outside health care, from Japanese and American industry. Common questions posed to all consultants were "Does it work?" and that question's corollary, "Does it work in health care?"

The National Demonstration Project, described in *Curing Health Care* (Berwick, Godfrey, & Roessner, 1990), was an excellent resource for beginning to address that issue. The project addressed the need for a changed approach to ensuring quality in health care. *Curing Health Care* describes many of the tools of TQI and recounts the TQI successes of pioneering health care institutions. The authors commented, "In the National Demonstration Project, the institutions represented at the outset by their chief executive or another top manager achieved the greatest success; those whose senior leaders were absent became the most frustrated" (p. 158).

During the implementation of TQI in VHA, top management at VA hospitals consisted of a director (chief executive officer), a chief of staff (a full-time physician and leader of the clinical staff), and an associate facility director. Some hospitals also had a head nursing executive, and larger facilities had an assistant facility director at the time of the initial TQI implementation.

Many writers and clinicians, from Deming and Juran to many others, have addressed the importance of leadership. Gaucher and

Coffey (1993) enumerate what they believe to be the key leadership characteristics required for a successful TQI effort. Of these attributes, VHA's TQI implementation planners implicitly or directly expected VA hospital leaders to exhibit at least the following:

- Ability to be customer-driven
- Ability to be a change agent
- Ability to manage uncertainty
- Visibility in the change process
- Commitment to education and training
- Willingness to delegate and decentralize decision making.

The pilot program did not call for, expect, or mandate significant activity from top management in areas such as

- Social activism outside the community of veterans (of course, many VA hospital managers are active in their community anyway, but such activity was not a part of the TQI program's expectations)
- Being or becoming a visionary
- Being people-oriented
- Commitment to innovation
- Capacity for introspection
- Openness to sharing information or fostering close relationships with suppliers

Although not required, these particular characteristics were recognized as valuable and worthwhile.

VHA's pilot effort in TQI emphasized the need to measure progress in terms of customer satisfaction. In the parlance of the consultant, VHA dealt with internal customers (other employees) and external customers (generally the patients being treated by the hospital and their family members). As called for by the implementation process, both sets of customers were surveyed early in each individual facility's implementation effort, and the resultant data were used to determine major areas of need. Hospital directors were supportive and participative in this process in virtually every facility, and the information gained was generally used to focus on real instances of hospital failure to meet customer expectations.

Hospital directors were clearly expected to act as change agents in the implementation effort. Many of the hospitals were blessed with actively involved leaders, in both the administrative and clinical staffs. The overall degree of involvement and participation in TQI activities—assessment activities and team membership mostly—was clearly related to the active involvement of the director and other members of top management. And in hospitals with visible, supportive management, the time from assessment to initial team formation and recommendations was considerably shorter than in facilities lacking adequate management participation.

The ability to manage uncertainty may be one of the greatest strengths of VHA's hospital directors as they deal each year with a fixed budget (often of an unknown amount until virtually the beginning of the fiscal year—October 1 in the federal government). The Department of Veterans Affairs has dealt, for the past decade, with decreasing budgets in the face of rising health care costs, particularly in the areas of personnel and technology. Further, as a political entity and a cabinet-level department, VA faces the usual changing of political agendas and priorities from year to year. The impact of these changes affects every level of the organization, for politics, like health care, is always local. The lack of certainty attached to participation in the TQI pilot was not of sufficient magnitude to cause any of the thirty-eight pilot facilities to withdraw or even complain (more than usual) about the circumstances, however.

VHA has never enjoyed congressional largesse in securing funding to train and educate its workforce. Some funding was available for training and education, for both top management and frontline employees, specifically tied to the TQI effort, however. The directors and chiefs of staff throughout the system were surveyed to determine their attitudes and beliefs about various aspects of TQI; the survey disclosed a recognition of the time commitment, including personal time, required for involvement and education in TQI processes (Al-Assaf and others, 1993; Tindill, Al-Assaf, & Gentling, 1993).

VHA's TQI implementation methodology included a clear expectation that hospital directors and other top management would delegate the proper level of authority to process owners to execute changes in their arena. As with the other implementation areas mentioned above, variations occurred in the degree and depth to which such authority was actually delegated. In those hospitals with a greater degree of delegation, there seemed to be more employee involvement in the process than there was in hospitals where the authority to make process changes was maintained at higher levels of the organization.

During the period of time covered by Phase II of the implementation pilot, twelve of the twenty-five facilities had a change in director. Even where the new director was an enthusiastic supporter of TQI and intended to be as supportive as his or her predecessor, there was usually a lag between the time the first director left and the other arrived, and an unavoidable loss of momentum occurred. A new director needs a certain amount of time to understand the culture and personnel of the facility well enough to be comfortable with delegating authority. In that same vein, employees are likely to withhold their active participation in a TQI change process while waiting to see if the new director is interested or involved in it.

Given the importance of the visible involvement of top management and the delegation of authority that can come only with familiarity, it should not be surprising that a comparison of the results of the TQI implementation between hospitals with stable leadership and those with turnover in directors during Phase II showed some striking differences. Of the facilities without any change in directorship, five won national recognition with a Robert W. Carey Quality Award. The Carey award is named for the late director of the Philadelphia regional benefits office, who was the driving force in making improvements in that office's customer service and benefits delivery. Annually, VA offices and facilities apply for the award by answering a self-administered assessment closely tailored to the Baldrige assessment. After review, some applicants are chosen for site visits, and a more rigorous evaluation is done. Winners are clearly high-performing organizations with obvious attention to customer service, employee involvement, and high-quality outcomes in an environment of continuous improvement. The fact that five of the twelve facilities that had consistent leadership in Phase II received recognition indicates some relationship between the two circumstances. That indication is strengthened by the fact that none of the thirteen facilities that had a change in directorship have received a Carey award. Another of the twelve facilities with consistent leadership, the VA hospital in Togus, Maine, applied for the prestigious Malcolm Baldrige Quality Award in Health Care, a pilot program in 1995, and was selected as a semifinalist. The picture is clear—consistent leadership, especially that which meets the characteristics listed by Gaucher and Coffey, leads to significant penetration of TQI into the organization, a high level of involvement of employees, and improved customer service, satisfaction, and outcomes.

One of the most obvious responsibilities of TQI pilot hospital's leadership was to define the facility's organizational mission, vision, and values. In *Curing Health Care*, the authors state that "the first task in quality improvement is clarification of the mission, and the second is commitment to change. Both require leadership. . . . When physician leadership and organizational leadership are separate, as they are in many hospitals, then the same requirement for commitment applies to both" (p. 157). Thus VHA's implementation plan included, as one of the key early responsibilities of top management, the drafting of a mission statement for each participating hospital. The Department of Veterans Affairs has a national mission statement that applies to its entire health care system; the TQI implementation plan indicated that the pilot hospitals' mission statements should be consistent with this national mission, which can be summarized as follows:

- Deliver the highest quality care
- Provide excellent educational opportunities for veterans through the department's academic affiliations
- Be involved in important biomedical and health services research
- Provide backup to the Department of Defense (DoD) in a national emergency

Atchison (1990) has stressed that in health care organizations there is a need for the leadership to create and sustain a strong culture through the definition and communication of the organizational mission, vision, and values as often as possible and through as many channels as can be found. Similarly, Nanus (1992) outlined four major leadership roles, placing primacy upon being a "direction setter" responsible for selecting and articulating organizational goals.

A mission statement is defined as a clear, concise statement of what an organization does (or should be doing) in terms of providing products or services and serving customers. An organizational vision describes the desired "future state" of an organization, including what others will be saying about it and about its products and services. A value statement articulates a clear set of organizational values that will guide the actions of everyone in the organization—as a shared behavior model—as they close the gap between the current mission and the future vision.

The methods used by the different pilot hospitals in creating their mission, vision, and value (MVV) statements varied but shared many features; the means of communicating the statements to employees also shared commonality but had a different flavor in each individual hospital. In most hospitals, the first drafts of the MVV statements were written by a high-level executive body such as the hospital quality steering committee or quality leadership team. The top management at the Tuscaloosa VA hospital drafted their MVV statement at a management retreat. In each hospital, although top management was involved and often directed the development of the MVV statement, it did not act alone. The usual practice, after top executives successfully define an organization's mission, vision, and values, is to issue a memorandum or communique to the organization's employees announcing the fact. Likewise, the pilot program emphasized the need for MVV statements to be shared throughout the facilities; there is no point to leadership's leaving such an important document in a vacuum. Japanese practitioners of TQI comment that the process of developing a common vision and understanding organizational mission is like growing a tree—it is a natural process that cannot be rushed and often takes years to complete. In a health care setting like a VA hospital or clinic, such an undertaking requires particular effort to ensure that all employees have an opportunity to comment and participate in the development of the statement.

Vision is an overarching construct that can provide energy, dedication, and commitment to a shared enterprise. The construct has a long history in many cultures, and it is mentioned in writings from as early as 1000 B.C. ("where there is no vision the people perish" [Prov. 29:18]) to the present (works by Stephen Covey [1989] and Peter Senge [1990], for example). Visions that have transformed society are familiar stories to many of us today: Alexander Graham Bell's vision of universal communication and Henry Ford's vision of universal automobile ownership. John Kennedy inspired a nation by setting before us a vision of placing a man on the moon by the end of the 1960s. That kind of vision lifts our heads; it is an important force in the human heart and mind that motivates us toward a higher purpose. A shared vision binds the people of an organization together and helps them strive toward achieving a common goal.

It is important to have the widespread endorsement and understanding of the workforce, both for the organization's mission and for its vision. Lyndon Johnson told of a visit he made to the Kennedy Space Center for a high-level ceremony. After the public festivities, the president, walking back through an empty hangar, encountered a man sweeping the floor. He asked him what his job was, and the man with the broom responded, "I am helping to put a man on the moon." That kind of understanding, personal acceptance, and involvement does not result from posting newly minted MVV statements on hospital bulletin boards. Effective vision cannot be imposed from above.

In the TQI pilot hospitals, there were two predominant methods of circulating draft MVV statements to the workforce for comment. One was to use the existing administrative structure in the various departments to cascade the document down through the organization. In this method, the department heads (or service chiefs, as they are called in VA hospitals) were expected to initiate the cascade and to collect comments for relaying back to top management for inclusion in revisions. In the other method, top management took the responsibility upon themselves to disseminate the draft MVV directly to employees, using newsletters, bulletin boards, and flyers. The call for feedback and comment was obvious in each case, but neither method resulted in significant employee input. Most employee comments were in the vein of minor changes in wording, not substantive thoughts about the content. Nonetheless, the leadership at those facilities where substantive changes were recommended, such as the Cleveland and Dayton, Ohio, hospitals and the Columbus, Ohio, outpatient clinic, used those suggestions to make changes in the document before it was re-presented to employees.

Each of the facilities used at least one method to solicit employee feedback, and this took longer to accomplish than the old method of having top management draw up the MVV statement during a weekend retreat. Total time from the beginning of the process to the completion and publication of an MVV statement was almost always several months. (The Columbus, Ohio, outpatient clinic took about two months, but this facility had fewer employees than most of the hospitals.)

Communication of the final position on MVV was transmitted throughout the facility, often using the same methodology as before. The domiciliary at White City, Oregon, used multiple methods to disseminate its MVV statement. Top management there used the usual newsletters and bulletin boards but also held open forums with employees to allow discussion and two-way exchange. They posted the MVV statement in large frames in high-traffic areas around the facility and provided every employee with a laminated card containing it. Top management walked the facility regularly and discussed the MVV statement with employees. As Kurt Gundacker, the master trainer who assisted the White City facility in its training, said, "When the leadership pays this much attention to the mission, it really drives the organization." White City won the Robert W. Carey Quality Award in 1995.

Although the TQI implementation plan called for the facility mission statements to support the Department of Veterans Affairs mission statement, it did not require any particular type of wording. Review of twelve mission statements from the Phase I and II facilities shows two similarities. First, nine of the twelve directly mention their endorsement of at least three of the concepts in the departmental mission statement. Facilities like the Big Spring, Texas, VA hospital did not comment on education and research as part of their mission, and a few of the other facilities—including those in proximity to military facilities—did not specifically mention their backup role for the Department of Defense in times of national emergency.

Many of the mission statements contained items that were vague and global and hard to disagree with but also quite hard to internalize and treat as truly unique: "the San Diego Network provides comprehensive health care" (San Diego); "the delivery of high-quality comprehensive healthcare to veteran patients" Chicago, West Side); "our efforts are focused first and foremost on our patient needs and expectations" (Brooklyn); "provide patient care to eligible veterans" (Dallas). In a few of the facilities, top management recognized the need for greater specificity and took necessary steps to get the MVV statement more focused. At Portland, the director, Barry Bell, assessed the original mission statement as too vague. It read, "To provide excellent health care, using the abilities of all employees, supported by our commitment to education and research." After reworking, the mission statement of the Portland VA hospital now reads,

> To provide comprehensive care based on a primary care model for a local population in a defined area. To provide tertiary services to a broad-based population that is also served by other VAMCs [VA medical centers]. To market clinical programs to other health care providers, including the Department of Defense, Indian Health Services, and other providers, as the Veterans Health Administration regulations allow. To maintain our education and teaching role with Oregon Health Sciences University and allied health affiliates. To maintain excellence in research that integrates clinical needs and research inquiry to enhance the quality of health care delivery to veterans.

The increased length provides greater specificity and allows each member of the facility to use the mission statement to help guide their decisions about which of various courses they might follow.

The White City domiciliary's mission statement avoids generalities and focuses directly on the mission of that particular facility: "Serves as a national resource for eligible veterans, providing quality residential treatment in psychiatry, addictions, geriatrics, medicine, physical and vocational rehabilitation. Provides high-quality primary outpatient medical and mental health care to veterans living in the southern Oregon and northern California region. Strives in partnership with the veterans we serve, to optimize the therapeutic goal of social and vocational integration of the veterans into their community." Half of the mission statements reviewed from the twelve facilities had local specificity of the same nature as that produced by White City: "within Central Ohio"

(Columbus OPC); "to West Texas veterans" (Big Spring, Texas); "we value the large community in which we exist" (Dayton, Ohio); "It is our vision to be the medical center of choice for veterans and health care workers in Jackson and the surrounding community" (Jackson, Mississippi).

In a couple of the facilities, the process of developing a mission statement was approached as a "paper exercise" originally, and the attitude of top management and leadership was apparent to the rest of the organization. The result was a rather quick writing of the MVV statement, little feedback from employees, and a short cycle time to produce a final product for dissemination. In one of these facilities, the master trainer remarked that top management realized about a year later that the mission statement was important to their understanding of where they were going and what they should be doing. At that point, attention was given to addressing the need for restructuring the mission statement. This recognition of the value of the mission statement in accomplishing the goals of the facility represents a maturation of thought and experience within the leadership of the facility. That same type of maturation occurred in other facilities as well throughout Phases I and II and helped all employees understand the usefulness of the mission statement in making day-to-day decisions.

The role of top management in promulgating the MVV statement, the dissemination of the statement to all employees, the expectation that everyone know and operate according to its tenets, and the willingness to reevaluate the mission when the external situation changes are of paramount importance to the success of any facility's TQI plan. Harrington (1987) has stressed that when an improvement process fails, it can usually be blamed on management: management either misused the process; did not participate in it; believed that some employee, not management, was the problem; failed to make a long-term commitment; or did not make it part of the facility's regular activity. During the implementation of TQI in the thirty-eight VHA pilot sites, those facilities where top management was directly, visibly, and consistently involved in the development and follow-through of a mission statement experienced broad employee involvement and improvement in both processes and outcomes. These facilities have already been recognized within VHA as having the right kinds of leadership and demonstrating high-quality activities.

The lessons we learned during Phases I and II were not new to those already involved in bringing a new organization into the philosophy of continuous improvement. Certainly the lessons do not represent new knowledge (even for health care, a relative late-comer to total quality management). Once again, we saw the over-riding importance of active, involved leadership on the process of enlisting employee involvement and producing important im-provements in services and outcomes. Clearly the facilities with the greatest leadership involvement performed best and with the shortest cycle times. We were able to confirm the observations of others that consistent leadership involvement is essential; perhaps even more important than the knowledge and skill of top man-agement is their daily presence and expectations of quality enhancement. Drennan (1992) has emphasized that top man-agement's visible commitment to quality is evident in their use of their own time. When leaders spend their time in meetings, mak-ing special efforts, and paying attention to the quality improve-ment activities in their organization, they establish the real priority. In VHA's experience, we have seen again and again that these observations have merit and have tracked well with the ex-perience of hospitals and clinics, in terms of both internal im-provements and external recognition.

The behaviors and attitudes of leadership, both clinical and ad-ministrative, at these successful facilities should be used as models for other health care organizations within the Department of Vet-erans Affairs and throughout the nonfederal sector.

References

Al-Assaf, A. F., Tindill, B. S., Curtis, K., Gentling, S. J., McCaffree, D. R., & Wheeler, J. (1993). Perceptions of VA chiefs of staff on total qual-ity management implementation. *American Journal of Medical Qual-ity, 8,* 123–127.

Atchison, T. (1990). *Turning health care leadership around: Cultivating in-spired, empowered, and loyal followers.* San Francisco: Jossey-Bass.

Berwick, D. M., Godfrey, A. B., & Roessner, J. (1990). *Curing health care: New strategies for quality improvement.* San Francisco: Jossey-Bass.

Covey, S. R. (1989). *The seven habits of highly effective people.* New York: Simon & Schuster.

Drennan, D. (1992). *Transforming company culture.* New York: McGraw-Hill.

Gaucher, E., & Coffey, R. J. (1993). *Total quality in healthcare: From theory to practice.* San Francisco: Jossey-Bass.

Harrington, J. H. (1987). *The improvement process.* New York: McGraw-Hill.

Nanus, B. (1992). *Visionary leadership: Creating a compelling sense of direction for your organization.* San Francisco: Jossey-Bass.

Senge, P. (1990). *The fifth discipline: The art and practice of the learning organization.* New York: Doubleday.

Tindill, B. S., Al-Assaf, A. F., & Gentling, S. J. (1993). Total quality improvement: A study of veterans affairs medical center directors and QA coordinators. *American Journal of Medical Quality, 8,* 45–52.

Chapter Nine

Involving Mid-Level Managers and Supervisors

Sherry Treiber

The role played by middle managers in a private hospital's total quality improvement (TQI) effort is significant and critical to its success. Similarly, mid-level managers—department heads, assistant chiefs, and key supervisory staff—played a significant role during the initial stages of the TQI effort in the Veterans Health Administration (VHA), contributing to its many successes and learning valuable lessons from its failures. Numerous books and articles on quality improvement have stressed that the support of top management is essential for a successful implementation of TQI. The experience in VHA was no different. Once the leadership of a given hospital accepted their responsibility to become involved and to model the continuous improvement philosophy, the process began in earnest. Many leaders and other employees became swept up in the exciting opportunities this different approach to organizational development offered and wanted to quickly involve the entire workforce and immediately set the improvement cycle in motion.

Even though some leaders, particularly the executive assistants for TQI and other local TQI specialists, recognized early on that the middle managers' role was important, other priorities often prevented them from being sufficiently involved in the process. Much was said about why mid-level supervisors were the way they were and why they exhibited non-TQI behavior at times, but little was in place to help them change. The importance of providing appropriate, targeted support to this key group of employees was finally recognized—after varying amounts of angst and difficulty in obtaining progress without their assistance. The recognition of the critical need for their support led to a change in the original implementation plan to include education specifically aimed at the needs of mid-level managers. This chapter describes some of VHA's experiences training these managers and the lessons that were learned from them.

VHA began its total quality journey at a time when management in both the public and private sectors was undergoing fundamental changes. In many businesses and organizations, teams were assuming much of the decision-making responsibility traditionally reserved for managers because chain-of-command communications did not meet emerging standards for customer service. Some managers even found themselves outside the decision-making loop. Organizations were flattening the ratio between the number of managers and subordinates, thus creating a greater span of responsibility (and, sometimes, a feeling of loss of control) for those who remained. These changes created increasing pressures on middle managers. In short, they found themselves in complex, close, ever-shifting relationships with the people they managed. It now appears (correctly) to many middle managers that the rules of the game have changed dramatically.

New expectations call for mid-level managers to behave in new ways and to master skills they never needed in the past fifteen or twenty years of their career. Many find themselves unprepared. As Zandy, Leibowitz, Shore, and Schuman (1992) explain, "[Their] challenges have to do with combining certain traditional behaviors and skills such as analytical thinking and a bottom-line focus, with the ability to listen well, give useful feedback, and serve as coach and mentor to subordinates in order to enhance both their satisfaction and their performance on the job." At one VA hospital, a clinical division chief adopted a "holding" position and even made negative comments about TQI, suggesting that she simply intended to wait for the whole idea to disappear. When the hospital director became aware of these comments, he met with the chief and explained the hospital's mission regarding implementation of TQI and his expectation that its department chiefs would support the effort. The chief began to volunteer staff to serve on TQI teams and ultimately accepted a role as team leader herself.

The expectation of such changes was especially frustrating or intimidating to managers who had excelled under the traditional, command-and-control management system of the past fifty years. The military-like infrastructure that characterized the early years of VHA exerted a strong influence on the organizational structure and hierarchy it developed. The promise of eventual long-term gain for the organization provided little comfort to those most threatened by the changes—mid- to late-career managers who had learned to be successful under the old system. These individuals were personally threatened by a process that required significant personal change and threatened their safety net.

Early Resistance

The existing management patterns in VHA were firmly entrenched. Managers worked hard to reach their status, and they received recognition for their ability to "take charge." Many had sought management positions so that they could have more say in the decisions that were made, since the lower ranks had traditionally been limited in their ability to do so. Understandably, new changes imposed by the total quality philosophy were not readily embraced by such managers, who had struggled to reach their goal and were satisfied with their role in the old system and felt it was their turn to make the decisions. This institutionalized reluctance to participate was exacerbated as mid-level managers saw themselves left out of early TQI activities. As one manager put it, "I have worked all my life to get to this level of the organization, and now you are changing the rules and telling me that the people I supervise are better able to solve problems than I am."

In addition, misunderstandings arose and rumors spread that the purpose of TQI was to eliminate supervisory positions. These rumors were easily fed and readily believed, since VHA's TQI rollout coincided with the national focus on reducing the size of government in the early 1990s. Efforts to streamline government operations frequently focused on reducing the numbers of mid-level managers (and, as a result, increasing the breadth of control in government organizations). In 1993, the ratio of supervisors to workers in government was one to seven; the National Performance Review (1993) established the goal of increasing that ratio to one to fifteen. Thus it is not hard to understand why some mid-level managers concluded that reducing the workforce, not empowering it, was the real reason for the emphasis on TQI.

This feeling was compounded by the reality that real empowerment does significantly reduce the need for narrow spans of control; indeed, problems can occur if the mid-level workforce is not reduced following TQI implementation, simply because there is so much opportunity for meddling. Each of these considerations has been seen and dealt with in industrial settings where TQI has been implemented, but they still represent major barriers to the successful implementation of the concept in hospitals (Lewis, 1993).

It is not surprising, therefore, that a variety of problems began to surface as managers faced up to the changes occurring in TQI environments. For example, at some VA hospitals, frontline employees served on quality leadership teams (QLTs)—the groups charged with planning and coordinating the TQI rollout at each hospital. These frontline staff now enjoyed regular access to the hospital leadership and other key personnel, who in more traditional times would have been out of their reach. Such access to leadership was both unfamiliar and threatening to middle managers, as one manager made clear when he told a QLT member, "Just remember who does your performance review." In another hospital, a department chief with a traditional, autocratic management style was unable to deal with different roles in team settings; thus his department was unable to successfully participate in hospital-wide TQI activities until the chief retired.

Disguised threats made by middle managers were accompanied by a host of other subtle manipulations designed to reinforce their position. Some managers rearranged employees' schedules to block their participation in TQI and played the "work load demands" trump card to justify their actions. Others showed an unwillingness to shift work loads, causing significant stress for employees trying to participate in TQI. Reports of supervisors' verbal and nonverbal discouragement of employee participation surfaced on a regular basis. Some comments were as blatant as, "Why are you wasting your time on that? TQI will never work around here." Others were more subtle but equally powerful:

"You'll need to cancel your TQI meeting today; the unit is too busy."

"If you want to be on that TQI team now, you will have to give up some of your other involvements."

"How long is this going to go on?"

"We have more important things than TQI to do around here today."

In one VA hospital, the lack of support from an important mid-level manager and that manager's refusal to allow team members time to attend TQI meetings caused the team activities to drag on for almost eighteen months before finally approaching conclusion. As a result, the individual members lost their enthusiasm for the project and the process.

One of the more interesting tactics used to block participation was revealed in this statement from a mid-level manager: "I don't say anything to promote TQI because I do not want to alienate one of the employees who does not believe in it." Other managers used time-honored passive-aggressive tactics like frowning, making heavy sighs, or shaking their head when employees attended TQI activities or talked about it. Some managers withheld information from team members, like a cook who shares a famous recipe but leaves out some of the ingredients so no one else can make quite as wonderful a concoction. Sometimes managers even erected barriers beyond their own sphere of influence. For example, one team needed some data from another department to complete a process assessment, but the supervisor in that department would not share the information until ordered to do so by the hospital director.

There were many reasons for such resistance (most of them related to VHA's management culture):

- Coaching was not supported or promoted.
- A lack of rewards and recognition provided few incentives to change.
- Top management did not act as role models or model TQI principles.
- Middle management was poorly educated on the benefits of TQI.
- Middle managers lacked time (crisis management was the norm).

- Middle managers lacked training in implementing TQI.
- Some managers had negative attitudes.
- Some managers were afraid.

In some cases, the organizational climate simply did not support or promote a coaching style: managers were not given the time or guidance they needed to mentor those who worked for them, and coaching efforts were not recognized or rewarded. In fact, most rewards and recognition reinforced traditional management practices, offering managers little incentive to change. At some VHA facilities, top leadership did not act as TQI role models or encourage the change to a new management style. At one VA hospital, when the QLT became aware of the degree of resistance to TQI implementation among department heads and key supervisors, they determined to "fix" the problem immediately using the time-honored method they had learned in the past—they would set everyone straight right away with a memorandum telling them how to act in the future!

This failure to model the appropriate behaviors reinforced the resistance of middle managers. Many managers did not receive education to help them recognize the benefits of the change and, most importantly, answer the question "what's in it for me?" Even when the benefits were clear, training often was not offered to middle managers to show them how to manage differently. Crisis management often prevailed—managers lacked the time to work on bringing about change—and fear of the unknown was widespread. With the many reasons for managers to behave the way they did, it was clear they would need more and better reasons to change and support TQI.

Changing Roles

In the early phases of TQI implementation, every level of the VHA system had a steep learning curve to discover what TQI was all about and how it was going to fit into their part of the organization. The focus was on planning, coordinating, and assimilating the concepts and principles of TQI into each of the Phase I and Phase II hospitals and on learning as much as possible from those experiences. As described earlier, change was tackled at all levels:

leaders were learning and trying on different leadership behaviors; education and training was initiated for all employees; and employee expectations were shifting. An infrastructure to support TQI had begun to develop, and the full impact and scope of this journey was understood in varying degrees.

This was a period of great excitement and apprehension. Significant change was long overdue, and finally a path was offered to overcome many of the difficulties and barriers associated with past change efforts. But recognizing needs did not always lead to action. As noted above, middle managers were known to be an important group for the success of TQI change efforts, but appropriate and necessary training for them was often delayed while competing priorities such as hospital-wide assessments, awareness training for all employees, and team and facilitator training captured the attention of the leadership and TQI personnel. As TQI moved ahead, unprepared middle managers felt the squeeze. Ann Sammons, chief of dietetics at the Prescott VA hospital, explained, "The supervisors are feeling tremendous pressure and treated like the bad guys around here. They are told to accomplish opposing priorities: 'serve the meals and support TQI data gathering activities'—that cannot be done when you are short-staffed. It's not an easy position to be in."

So, as TQI was introduced in VA hospitals, the middle manager raised many questions: "What will happen to me? Where do I fit in? Why *should* I change? What am I supposed to do?" Some facilities held special classes for supervisors and managers to address these concerns. However, this type of intervention was usually limited to basic information and did not provide the structure and follow-up to accomplish real change in management roles. The Dayton VA hospital recognized the need and the lack of a ready answer from within VHA, so they used an outside consultant specifically to train their mid-level managers about how to become "enlightened leaders" and active participants in the implementation process.

In this early stage of the system's TQI implementation, changes in middle management behavior depended heavily on role modeling from leaders, particularly top leaders. Some hospital directors possessed a leadership style that fit easily with TQI culture and clearly demonstrated to others what was expected. Other directors accepted the challenge of changing their style and recognized that it would require time and persistence. In many of these facilities the middle managers were not quick to fall in line; they were content to wait and see if the changes in the management style and decision-making methods of the director were real before they got involved themselves. Whatever the outcome, this informal approach was often the beginning step in the management transition.

A number of miscellaneous activities were attempted at various hospitals to include middle managers in the TQI effort and get their endorsement and involvement. Some were invited to become involved at the level of the process improvement team as leaders, facilitators, or members. This participation gave them a direct means of understanding and practicing TQI methods. Some became TQI trainers and established themselves as facility experts. Also, many QLTs had representatives from the ranks of middle management. Various reward and recognition efforts were implemented to reinforce middle managers' support of TQI initiatives; these were often in the form of a variety of formal and informal thank-yous. In rare cases, TQI participation became an expected and explicit part of a manager's performance standard.

These methods were not systematic or widespread, but positive outcomes were noticeable where they existed. Some department heads became noted champions of the TQI philosophy; Gary Abreu, chief of engineering at the Dayton VA hospital, and James Carey, chief of pharmacy, actively chartered many teams within their departments and actively supported them. One hospital began its implementation using mid-level managers almost exclusively as trainers. Years later, these individuals still maintain direct participation in TQI activities throughout the hospital.

A more formal aspect of the implementation process also began to produce favorable results in pockets of the organization. Individual department-level implementations, or "service quality deployments," had the most significant impact on changing middle managers' roles, particularly for those who already had a natural tendency toward a participative management style. These department-level TQI efforts provided a structured, team approach to planning, prioritizing, and taking action, and they offered the department heads a specific TQI role as leader of the effort. But there were persistent cries across the system for more training and involvement than could be produced at the local level. These concerns and requests for support from the national level grew louder and were finally recognized as time went by. Something else was needed to truly guide middle managers into new skills and behaviors.

Finally, in the fall of 1993, an education course was made available to specifically address this gap in management support. "Coaching and Mentoring Skills for Managers and Supervisors" was designed by the TQI training staff at VHA's continuing education center as a five-day course to be presented over several months.

It would have been extremely helpful had this course or one like it been available in the early phases, because it addressed several crucial needs. First, it would have drawn closer attention to the middle managers and provided the structure and support that many sought during those transitional times. Facilities that initiated this course reported very positive results. Don Gray, an executive assistant for TQI, described some of the benefits: "The course was designed for the participants to put the concepts and ideas into action with the help and support of peer mentors. Through this experience some managers actually became more involved and invested in TQI; and it became an excellent forum for managers to discuss issues and concerns together." Mike Blathers, chief of the security department at a VA hospital, offered his own impression after participating in the course: "This course gave me a practical, hands-on approach and reinforced many of my own ideas. It forced me to look at my style of managing in a much different way than what I learned in college. Our managers are now fostering a team spirit and giving employees more say and ownership in what is happening around here. It is definitely something that supervisors and managers benefit from, especially as employees are becoming more diverse."

Lessons Learned

Looking back on the first years of TQI in VHA, it is easy to say that involving managers and supervisors was not our greatest accomplishment. However, a major strength built into the implementation process was an emphasis on continuously searching for those aspects of TQI implementation that worked well and for those that required further attention. VHA's experience reinforced the concept that a systems approach for addressing management role changes is necessary and is particularly beneficial in the early stages of a TQI implementation effort.

Certain lessons or strategies can be taken from this experience. These are described below and summarized in Exhibit 9.1.

The following points are particularly important:

1. *Active involvement of mid-level managers is critical.* In order to ensure that mangers are involved and productive in the TQI process, several key steps must be taken: first, someone or some group must accept responsibility for addressing mid-level management involvement. Just as the involvement of physicians is key to accomplishing the anticipated benefits of TQI, so is the participation of key administrative supervisors. Whoever accepts this responsibility, whether the QLT, an existing supervisory council, or a newly chartered process improvement team, must develop and carry out plans for monitoring managerial involvement. Second,

Exhibit 9.1. Lessons Learned.

- Identify the group responsible for addressing TQI.
- Assess current management's role in the organization and what exists to support the change.
- Define and communicate how you *really* want people to behave.
- Develop an action plan:

  Identify specific behaviors to be modeled by top leadership and other key personnel.

  Identify and build manager stakeholders in the process (establish the "critical few").

  Identify and use managers as TQI trainers, team leaders, and/or facilitators.

  Provide specific training to introduce new skills and role alternatives.

  Use concrete methods to reward and recognize middle managers for desired behaviors and changes.

  Focus on continuous, small doses—continuously rewarding, recognizing, and reinforcing TQI behavior.

there must be educational and training efforts aimed at the specific needs of this very important group of employees. Recognition of national issues such as job security are important, but it is more important to focus on the actual concerns of local managers in developing and presenting training and information. Also, importantly, there must be a change in the local reward and recognition system to provide continual motivation for mid-level managers to be involved in and successful with the TQI program. This may mean completely rewriting the performance rating system or just developing a meaningful way to recognize the role played by middle managers in the improvements seen throughout the hospital and the system. Whatever the assigned accountability, long-term success depends upon how effectively this issue is addressed and how completely managers are included in the implementation loop.

2.   *Assess current management involvement, barriers, and opportunities.* As mentioned earlier, TQI implementation efforts did not often attend to or adjust the existing functions that shaped and supported management attitudes. Knowledge of the current situation is important, including the status of managers within the facility (their self-image, ability to make key decisions, training needs, and so on). This will help identify the priorities necessary to facilitate changes. Some questions to ask include the following:

What level of participation exists in the current organizational culture? Are all employees involved in decision making?

Are command-and-control systems the norm?

Are there barriers to the participation of frontline workers? Are there barriers to the participation of managers?

What level of authority do managers have now—what decisions *can* they make? Are they using this authority?

What level of group problem solving do managers allow?

What tools do managers use with their teams? Are they proficient in the use of these tools?

What systems are in place to discourage or encourage the changes necessary for TQI implementation (such as public recognition, performance appraisals, and so on)?

What system for accountability is in place to ensure that managers lead teams? What measures exist to determine if teams are effective in their department?

What management training and development opportunities are available to support the desired changes? Which have been utilized? Are they effective?

3.   *Define and communicate how you really want people to behave.* It is essential for the leadership's actions to match its statements of expectations. Whatever values are chosen as important and whatever actions are considered necessary should be modeled daily by the leadership, and that same expectation should be extended to mid-level managers. What this means on a day-to-day basis must be recognized and built into the activities of all involved in the implementation.

4.   *Develop an action plan.* VHA's TQI experience reinforced the notion that middle managers are in a critical position to support or thwart organizational change efforts. A systematic, planned approach can make the difference, ensuring that their influence is positive and their voices heard within each change activity. From successes and failures during the early stages of TQI implementation, various actions were identified that supported middle manager involvement. Modeling specific, desirable behaviors by top leadership and other key personnel exerted a significant impact. Middle manager stakeholders were identified and built up, thereby establishing the "critical few" within the change process. Middle managers were used successfully as TQI trainers, team leaders, and facilitators to assist their understanding, participation, and promotion of TQI principles. Concrete methods of rewarding and recognizing this group for desired behaviors and changes were established in various areas and degrees. This was a strong tool for reinforcing the TQI efforts that managers were making within the process, particularly when provided in continuous, small doses. And although its use was limited in the early implementation phases, specific training to introduce new skills and alternative roles was identified as important for addressing this group's unique challenges and needs.

The above strategies will support individual growth and change across a facility, but many *organizational* growth issues must be addressed simultaneously by top leadership for any lasting change to occur. These include the following:

- Sharing an understandable vision
- Allowing risk taking and mistakes
- Creating feedback systems that work
- Building a trusting environment
- Understanding and capitalizing on diversity
- Developing confidence in others, to allow real change

As discussed elsewhere, these organizational growth issues relate to what leadership promotes in the environment and culture that allows change to begin and grow. These efforts need to be intentional and unwavering.

Sharing an understandable vision of the future throughout the organization is especially important. Such a vision provides a focal point for employees, helping them work together toward achieving a common goal. Another important strategy is to allow risk taking and mistakes. Many of the most significant TQI lessons learned have resulted from our mistakes over the past several years. Conversely, fear and avoidance of risk has been one of our greatest barriers to change. The importance of leadership's permission to take calculated risks and make mistakes cannot be overstated. This also enhances the leadership's ability to build an organization where trust and change can be nurtured.

Another important organizational growth issue is the ability to understand and capitalize on diversity. A wealth of ideas and creativity has surfaced from the various groups and organizational levels that exist throughout the VA health care system. Lastly, leadership's confidence in others is the mark of true change. This is a particular struggle for those leaders who are used to more traditional management techniques and are changing past behaviors to match a new organizational direction. VHA leaders attempting this have been initially viewed with a good deal of skepticism, which only their constancy and persistence have overcome.

The involvement of middle managers is essential to the successful implementation of TQI. They are key to supporting the development and participation of frontline employees within the new organizational climate and for communicating and sharing leadership's priorities for the future. In the initial phases of TQI implementation in VHA, it quickly became apparent where, how, and to what extent this group impacted the overall effort. We have already taken significant steps forward in learning new middle management priorities, and we are well prepared to continue this path as we continue our total quality journey.

Conclusion: Involving Middle Managers at Prescott

Early TQI implementation efforts were replete with excitement, enthusiasm—and inexperience. The leadership of the Prescott VA hospital volunteered to participate in this fledgling effort and gained insights early on into the importance of involving middle managers. The TQI rollout at Prescott was fairly typical of the Phase One pilot sites.

The medical center's director had been the leader at Prescott for five years. He was known for his management style of strong control, solitary decision making, and personal vision. Middle management skepticism was voiced right away—not believing that an organizational change would really take place, that the director would really promote empowerment, and that they would be expected to participate. Initial training efforts targeted the top leadership, physicians, and a handful of key personnel to obtain initial understanding and "buy-in." This was immediately followed by a sweeping effort to provide awareness training to all employees as their introduction to what was coming. Special awareness sessions were developed for supervisors and managers, with an extra hour built in to discuss issues of changing roles and management concerns.

A TQI strategic plan was designed, and the first TQI teams were launched. Membership on these teams was determined by willingness, enthusiasm, knowledge of the process, and key service representation. This, by chance, included several mid-level managers who served in leadership roles, as facilitators, or as team members. The first year of implementation saw an expanding number of process improvement teams, and "service quality deployments" were initiated in those departments that were interested. But once the initial fanfare died down, management issues began to surface in earnest. Those managers who initially believed the facility leaders would falter began to realize that the changes were not going away, and frustrations mounted. In response, they remained diligent in their efforts to identify and describe all inconsistencies in others' behavior during this transitional time. The facility's emphasis during this stage was on voluntary participation from all levels of the organization—no one was forced or coerced. Volunteers were not in short supply, but middle management roadblocks were becoming more pronounced. Some employees reported feelings of "TQI harassment" when they tried to get involved, and a wide range of barriers kept surfacing.

It was becoming clear that middle manager support was a critical link for ongoing success and the accomplishment of true organizational change. Managers who were supportive and involved generated greater employee involvement and eagerness for change. Therefore, efforts were expanded to reward and recognize the supportive efforts of middle managers, to include more middle managers on teams, and to invite their participation in more of the TQI training activities. Top leadership was also making consistent attempts to share their expectations for how managers needed to behave in the TQI environment. A management retreat introduced empowerment principles, training, and planning.

All of the management interventions used in the first two years of implementation were sporadic and generally inconsistent. But as experience and awareness of what worked and did not work grew, a clearer plan and focus began to evolve. It was evident, however, that an earlier strategy that anticipated middle manager needs would have prevented many problems for managers and employees alike.

References:

Lewis, A. (1993, March). Too many managers: Major threat to CQI in hospitals. *Quality Review Bulletin,* pp. 95–101.

National Performance Review. (1993). *Streamlining management control* (pp. 9–13). Washington, DC: U.S. Government Printing Office.

Zandy, B., Leibowitz, J., Shore, E., & Schuman, G. M. (1992, March). Managers can be developers too. *Training & Development.*

Chapter Ten

Assessing Organizational Needs and Customer Expectations

John P. Morrison

Many organizations are attempting to create an environment in which continuous improvement becomes a natural part of conducting business. To be successful in meeting this challenge, organizations must first determine the needs of their customers. An organizational assessment is a valuable tool for gathering this information. It involves gaining an understanding of customers' expectations and their perceptions of quality. Products must possess the physical characteristics the customer desires and provide the functionality the customer expects. Services are judged differently, however. The customer's perception of quality may involve more than the service itself—it often includes the manner and the environment in which the service is provided. During recent years, the health care industry has experienced many changes in the way it provides services as a result of customer expectations. In fact, many of today's hospitals have developed hotel-like environments, including valet parking, bellboys, and curbside admissions.

Organizations can gain an understanding of their customers' expectations and perceptions of quality in a number of ways. A common technique is to use some form of customer satisfaction survey. In the not-too-distant past, knowing what the customer wanted and using that knowledge was sufficient to ensure success for most organizations. However, in today's competitive environment, simply doing what the customer wants is no longer enough. Competition requires that the customer's expectations be not only met but exceeded—and that this be accomplished quickly and efficiently.

To meet the demands of a highly competitive environment, organizations must continuously improve every facet of their operation. To accomplish this, organizations must have a thorough understanding of their operations and internal environment, know their strengths and weaknesses, and have a method for identifying opportunities for improvement. A strategy for determining whether improvement initiatives have been successful is also critical. In other words, they need to continuously assess their organization. This process is commonly referred to as organizational self-assessment.

There are some common characteristics of organizational assessments. First, they focus primarily on the perceptions of the internal customer, the employees who are responsible for developing the product or providing the service to the external customer. While the external customer determines what the end product or service will be, it is the internal customer who determines how the organization will produce the product or provide the service. Thus their needs and perceptions are critical to the efficient production of the final product or service. Second, an organizational assessment reviews all elements of the organization. This usually involves leadership, information and analysis, strategic quality planning, human resources, quality assurance activities, end results (that is, the final product or service), and customer satisfaction. Third, assessments are used to provide information for the continuous improvement process. Normally the first assessment establishes baseline data by which future assessments can be measured; this helps in determining what areas have experienced improvement and what areas are in need of further attention. And last, all internal customers are encouraged to participate in the assessment process.

Organizational Assessments

In 1991, when the Veterans Health Administration (VHA) committed itself to total quality improvement (TQI), it recognized that an important part of developing a TQI organization is continuous improvement. To continuously improve its organizations, VHA needed to continuously assess them. To do this it developed a system of continuous feedback, not only from external customers but also from internal customers.

Although VHA had a wealth of experience gathering feedback from external customers, it did not possess organizational tools for obtaining information from internal customers. Therefore VHA found it necessary to rely on a consulting firm that had some expertise in developing organizational assessment tools. In the fall of 1991, VHA, with the assistance of the American Productivity and Quality Center (APQC) consulting firm, developed its first organizational assessment tool.

TQI Assessment

VHA's TQI assessment tool was essentially based on the seven examination categories of the Malcolm Baldrige National Quality Award:

1. Leadership
2. Information and analysis
3. Strategic quality planning
4. Human resources
5. Quality assurance of products and services
6. Quality results
7. Customer satisfaction

The tool was designed for use by each VA hospital as part of its individual TQI initiative. The goal was to assess the quality of major processes in the hospital, as well as customer satisfaction. The assessment would permit each hospital to identify its strengths as well as opportunities for improvement. In essence, it was designed to give the hospitals a starting point for launching process improvement teams.

Case Study

The VA hospital in Oklahoma City was one of the initial Phase I pilot sites. They conducted their initial assessment from October through December 1991. The assessment process consisted of four parts: selection of team members, team training and organization, data collection, and wrap-up.

One of the first tasks of the hospital's steering committee was to establish the assessment team. This team of twenty-nine individuals was mostly composed of the senior leadership, department heads (both clinicians and administrative staff), and administrative officers. The team was then divided into eleven subteams for more effective assessment of specific areas:

1. Leadership
2. Information and analysis
3. Strategic quality planning
4. Human resources utilization
5. Quality assurance (health care providers)
6. Quality assurance (patients)
7. Quality results (health care providers)
8. Quality results (patients)
9. Quality results (affiliated customers)
10. Customer satisfaction (health care providers)
11. Customer satisfaction (patients)

The subteams were composed of three to five people. Several members served on more than one team.

Once the team members were assigned, they received two days of training and attended a planning meeting. The training, which was conducted by hired consultants, focused on data collection and various methods for obtaining the information needed to conduct the assessment. Also at this meeting, each of the subteams developed a strategy for obtaining information.

During the third part of the assessment, which took approximately six weeks, the team gathered their data and wrote a report of their findings. The information for their findings was primarily obtained through historical data, interviews, and surveys (both written and oral).

In early December, the assessment team came together for the fourth and final part of the assessment, a one-day wrap-up where each of the eleven teams presented its findings to the group. Based on the information presented, the assessment team identified fifty-three opportunities for improvement. They then used a nominal group process to prioritize them. A final document was assembled and presented to the hospital quality leadership team for action.

Recognizing the need to focus on high-priority processes, the hospital quality leadership team met to determine which of the fifty-three opportunities they would attempt to improve through the use of process improvement teams. The criteria they used for selecting opportunities were as follows:

1. Is the opportunity for improvement highly visible?
2. Is there ample opportunity for improvement?
3. Will the team be able to improve the process quickly?

Four of the five processes chosen were listed in the top eight of the prioritized list generated by the assessment process:

- Increase medical records availability
- Decrease the amount of waiting time in outpatient areas
- Institute a reward, recognition, and performance evaluation system
- Formalize patient education

A fifth opportunity for improvement—chosen but not listed as a high priority—was parking. This was done because of the high visibility of the parking issue and its impact on patients and staff.

Critique of the Assessment Tool

Although the initial assessment tool was found to be of value by those hospitals that chose to use it, it was recognized that it was cumbersome, difficult to use, and needed some changes. Some of the feedback from the hospitals included the following:

1. The tool itself was complex and difficult to use. After two days of training, many on the assessment team were still uncertain as to how they should obtain the information they needed.
2. The process was labor-intensive for the small number of staff who participated.
3. A very small segment, only 2 percent of the hospital staff, participated in administering the assessment.

4. Those who were involved were primarily management. Many questioned the validity of an assessment that involved only a few people, most of them top management.

5. Others questioned whether the results truly assessed the hospital, wondering if it were simply an elaborate means for justifying the selection of identified opportunities for improvement.

Quality System Survey

It was clear, based on the feedback from the pilot sites, that many hospitals wanted a simpler assessment tool. As a result, VHA put together a team of experienced TQI practitioners to revise the tool. The team included Steve Gentling, director at the Oklahoma City VA hospital; Steve Orwig, associate chief of staff for education at Oklahoma City; Darryl Heustis, chief of staff at the Loma Linda VA hospital; Galen Barbour, associate chief medical director for quality management; and Barbour's deputy, Frank Citro. The team also included hired consultants. In revising the initial tool, they addressed the key issues that had been raised earlier. The revised assessment tool had to correct the problems in the original assessment tool:

1. *Complexity:* The new tool had to be easy to administer and understand.
2. *Labor-intensiveness:* Assessments should require a relatively short time to complete.
3. *Participation:* Everyone should have the opportunity to participate.
4. *Validity:* The results should accurately reflect what the tool attempted to measure.

Fortunately, the team did not have to start from scratch. They were able to adapt an existing assessment instrument developed by the Pacer Group, which had subcontracted with the APQC consulting group to provide consulting services in VA hospitals. The Pacer instrument was designed for use in private industry, however, and some of its terminology was not appropriate for a health care setting. For example, one statement read, "The company president and his senior managers take an active part in promoting quality."

Such a statement was easily adapted to a VA hospital setting by changing it to read, "The director, chief of staff, and associate director take an active part in promoting quality." The revised tool was completed in November 1992. Like the earlier tool, this one was also modeled after the Malcolm Baldrige criteria. It addressed seven major categories:

- Management role
- Information and analysis
- Planning for quality
- Human resources utilization
- Quality assurance of products and services
- Quality results
- Patient satisfaction

The quality system survey (QSS) also asks seven questions focusing on demographic data. The QSS successfully meets the criteria established for it:

　　1. *Complexity.* Except for the demographics, the QSS is a standardized measurement tool. It uses variable data in describing participants' perceptions of a specific statement. To describe this perception, participants read a statement and then circle a number on a progressive scale to reflect their belief in the accuracy of the statement. For example, the first statement under "Management Role" is

　　The director, chief of staff, and associate director work hard to project an image of "quality first" to the general public.

Strongly Disagree　　　　　　　　　　　　　　　Strongly Agree
1　　　　2　　　　3　　　　4　　　　5　　　　6　　　　7

　　2. *Labor-intensiveness.* The QSS tool does not require participants to answer questions or respond to a statement in a narrative form. They simply read the statement and circle the response that most accurately reflects their perception. There are eighty-nine statements. The average person is able to complete the survey in twenty to thirty minutes.

3.   *Participation.* Unlike the first tool, all staff are given the opportunity to participate.

4.   *Validity.* In addition to the validity statements designed into the survey, it also contains other characteristics that increase its validity.

- Each of the eighty-nine statements are short and to the point, thereby decreasing the likelihood of subjectivity.
- All hospital staff are encouraged to participate in the survey. This increases the probability that the results will reflect the perceptions of the entire hospital, not just those of management.
- Participation is voluntary.
- The identity of the respondent is not requested. Participants are more likely to respond to a statement honestly when they are not required to identify themselves. Answer sheets are sealed in an envelope by the participant and mailed to the hospital's executive assistant for TQI. The results are tabulated and a report produced by a group outside the hospital.

Use of the QSS in Phase II

The QSS was first used in Phase II VA hospitals. The survey results were tabulated by Pacer Group staff, who generated a report for the hospitals. The report was divided into twelve sections. The first section was an executive summary. It provided an overview of the survey tool and of how the report was assembled, plus a brief summary of the hospital's assessment results. This included identified strengths as well as weaknesses. Section Two listed the survey responses with a mean score for each category. Section Three described the demographics of those staff who participated in the survey, categorized according to the following variables:

- Length of employment at VA facility
- Length of time in present position
- Level of position at the facility
- Level of contact with patients
- Primary beneficiaries of the respondent's work (patients, doctors, internal customers, and so on)
- Education level

Sections Four through Ten outlined the survey responses, breaking them down for each of the seven categories addressed by the survey (management role, information and analysis, planning for quality, human resources utilization, quality assurance of products and services, quality results, and patient satisfaction).

In addition to the improvements already mentioned, the QSS, unlike the initial tool, is standardized. Hospitals are able to compare their scores against other VA hospitals as well as against previous winners of the Baldrige award. Scores are provided for each question in the survey, as shown in Figure 10.1.

Section Eleven compares the hospital's scores against the Baldrige criteria. This is accomplished by giving an individual score for each of the seven categories and then an aggregate score to describe the overall culture of the hospital.

Section Twelve is a continuation of the demographics analysis. It outlines the percentage of staff from the various departments who participated in the survey.

Ownership of the QSS

During the Phase II rollout, the Pacer Group charged VHA $8,000 for each hospital to administer the QSS. Projecting that cost to the approximately 130 VA hospitals in Phases III and IV showed a potential cost of $1,040,000 over two years. That cost covered only first-time administration of the QSS and did not cover follow-up

Figure 10.1. QSS Score Format.

The director, chief of staff and associate director work hard to project an image of "quality first" to the general public.

Strongly Disagree					Strongly Agree	
1	2	3	4	5	6	7

Your Score _____ 5.2

Baldrige _____ 5.8

QSS Average _____ 5.1

surveys by individual hospitals. Because of that cost, VHA staff negotiated an agreement with the Pacer Group to purchase the QSS software and database for $40,000. The purchase agreement gave VHA complete rights to the QSS, including the right to administer the survey wherever and whenever it wanted to. Following Phase II, the QSS was administered by VHA staff at the St. Louis continuing education center.

Summary of the QSS

By 1995, over one hundred VA hospitals had used the QSS as one of their tools for assessing quality. As earlier stated, one of its primary advantages is that it is standardized. As such, it can be used as a tool not only for determining growth and change in processes but also for measuring change in the organizational culture. The initial QSS can serve as a baseline for measuring future change. It can be used not only to measure change in individual medical centers but also to measure change in the VA health care system as a whole.

The Robert W. Carey Quality Award

Another means for an organization to assess its improvement is to apply for quality awards. When applying for a quality award, an organization describes its quality improvement initiatives and their impact on its products or services. In addition, awards serve as a means for communicating and sharing quality outcomes and formally recognizing organizations that strive for excellence. In fact, many organizations today use the winners of national quality awards as benchmarks, since their processes are formally recognized as the best in current practice.

Another important factor concerning national quality awards is that the application process requires organizations to assess themselves. This assessment differs from organizational self-assessments such as the QSS, however. With self-assessments, organizations learn about their strengths and weaknesses. They gain an understanding of what needs to be improved. Quality award assessments, on the other hand, focus on quality improvement outcomes and descriptions of how the organization achieved them.

Nevertheless, when the award examiners review the application packages, they do not focus only on segments of the organization but instead try to view the organization as a whole. This includes how the organization improved its work processes and what it has done to improve its culture.

The leadership of VA recognized the value and need for a national quality award as a part of its TQI initiative. As a result, in 1993 they established the Robert W. Carey Quality Award. This award is dedicated to the memory of Robert W. Carey, who as director of the Veterans Affairs Regional Office and Insurance Center in Philadelphia, Pennsylvania, was recognized as a quality leader and a champion for excellence in the federal government.

The Robert W. Carey is an annual award. It currently has the following six eligibility categories:

- Health care
- Long-term health care
- Benefits services
- National cemeteries
- Support services
- United health care and benefits

From the six categories, one overall winner and one winner in each category is selected. All Department of Veterans Affairs organizations are eligible and encouraged to compete for the award. The award criteria embody the following fundamental concepts of TQI:

- Quality is defined by the customer.
- A TQI organization is driven by continuous improvement.
- The focus is on preventing errors rather than detecting them.
- Everyone participates in quality improvement.
- Senior management creates quality values and builds the values into the way the organization operates.
- Employees are valued and recognized for their involvement and accomplishments.
- Performance improvement is continuously measured.

The criteria are similar to those used for the Baldrige award. Department of Veterans Affairs organizations that have applied for the Robert W. Carey Quality Award have found the application process to be a valuable organizational assessment tool.

Lessons Learned

VHA began using organizational assessments in 1991. Since that time we have learned some valuable lessons about how to effectively use these tools for improving the efficiency and quality of the organization. Successful approaches to organizational assessments often share a number of common characteristics:

1. *They are multidimensional.* Organizational assessments need to be multidimensional. Our initial tool focused primarily on process outcomes. It was designed to tell us what processes we needed to improve to better meet the needs of our external customers. It did not focus on the needs of the internal customer. We have learned that focusing on improving the culture of the organization is a key ingredient in continuous improvement.

2. *They assess the organization's culture.* Organizational assessments need to capture the organization's culture. VHA's initial assessment tool was designed for the input of a few, and those few consisted of the leadership of the organization. For continuous improvement to become a part of the culture of an organization, everyone must participate.

3. *They can be used as working tools.* An organizational assessment needs be a working tool for continuous improvement. The first assessment should establish baseline data. Future assessments can then be used to identify improvements already accomplished and opportunities for further improvement. It will also identify trends.

4. *They are flexible.* Organizational assessments need to be flexible. There is a certain degree of trial and error in designing an assessment tool. The tool may have to be revised several times before it becomes an effective instrument. Also, VHA's environment and the expectations of its customers (both internal and external) are continuously changing. The assessment process needs to reflect those changes.

5. *They use multiple methods.* Finally, more than one method of assessment should be used. For example, VHA uses both the QSS and the Robert W. Carey award application process as organizational assessment tools.

Chapter Eleven

Implementing Training: A Phased Approach

R. W. Thomale Jr.

Training is the lifeblood of any growing, dynamic organization. As Vogt and Murrell (1990) point out, "Training is a distinct and vital dimension of today's workplace. It prepares people—human resources—to be more effective and efficient. If an organization is to develop into an empowering system, training must become a central focus of attention and effort. . . . Training cannot be relegated to second-class status and forced to subsist on budgetary leftovers." Although their comments apply to all training within an organization, they particularly apply to training designed to completely change an organization's culture—and this is what the Veterans Health Administration (VHA) was undertaking to do with its systemwide total quality improvement (TQI) training and rollout in the early 1990s.

Approaches to total quality training vary among consultants. Many have made themselves rich advocating the training of all employees on all or most elements of total quality before beginning implementation. This approach is intended to ensure that employees' fears do not overcome the process once implementation begins; after training, this approach holds, employees will be supportive, knowledgeable, and better able to make the implementation successful (Vogt & Murrell, 1990, p. 116). Such training is primarily classroom-based and theoretical in nature, although the better courses include practical exercises. It takes time to develop capable presenters; thus it is logical in such an implementation scheme for the consultants themselves to provide most, if not all, of the training. This becomes very expensive, however.

There is another training philosophy that embraces the belief that skills, techniques, and concepts learned in a classroom setting must be used in practical applications as a part of learning. To be most effective, the time between learning and applying what is learned must be as short as possible. Gitlow and Gitlow (1987) emphasize that linkage when they observe, "Once people are trained, they should be given the opportunity to use what they have learned as soon as possible. This will substantially reinforce their learning. If people have to wait to use what they have gained in training, they may forget a significant amount of information and/or skills" (p. 109). Athletic coaches know and apply this philosophy every day. After a classroom session, in which plays are discussed, assignments are presented, and overall play concepts are discussed, the team takes to the practice field; there what was learned in the classroom is put to immediate use. Plays are run again and again until the coach is satisfied that real learning has occurred. The classroom is reinforced with actual practice. Training in quality improvement skills is most successful when it is similarly reinforced. Training must be a tool to achieve results. Consultants Ernst and Young describe the use of that tool when they state, "The sooner the learning can be applied on the job, the better. Typically, if the concepts are not used within two weeks, the participants only remember the 'buzz words' and cannot competently apply the skills" (Ernst & Young Quality Improvement Consulting Group, 1990, pp. 105–106).

If before beginning its TQI implementation VHA had provided each employee with four to eight hours of awareness training, twenty-four to forty hours of leader/facilitator training, twenty-four to forty hours of team training, and so on, its TQI effort might have gone the way of management by objectives, zero-based budgeting, quality circles, and other strategies that focus on training rather than results. Such an investment of man-hours and dollars before obtaining tangible results probably would have doomed the process to the same kind of failure experienced by previous attempts to substantively change the organization's culture and operations. Having learned from unsuccessful "flavor-of-the-month" programs in the past, for its TQI implementation VHA chose to provide initial awareness training to all employees who were interested and then provide more specific training only as needed. This phased approach permitted the organization to develop training materials that were really VHA-oriented, to pilot those materials, and then to modify them based on input from VHA staff.

Early on, VHA planners were faced with a difficult decision. Mindful of Dr. Berwick's observation, "To meet the training needs, several organizations have chosen to build their own internal training resources, a costly and difficult undertaking that requires long-term commitment" (Berwick, Godfrey, & Roessner, 1990, p. 153), VHA decided it was less costly in the long run to develop in-house trainers than to be forever dependent on outside consultants. The choice was made to use the staff at the VHA's regional medical education centers (RMECs), scattered throughout the United States. The RMECs were staffed with trained educators whose duties were to provide educational offerings to the various hospitals, according to local need, and to develop and present programs of national interest as directed by the headquarters staff in the Office of Academic Affairs. The TQI implementation plan called for these educators to receive specific training from the external consultant, with the goal of ultimately replacing the external consultant with a well-trained cadre of mobile internal experts. This plan would save considerable amounts of money in each year of the implementation. The training of RMEC staff—to be known as master trainers—would be accomplished both in classroom settings as well as during the actual implementation at Phase I and II sites. The master trainers would help the paid consultants train staff at each VA hospital and, at the same time, develop their own skills, not only as trainers but also as consultants. At the completion of the first two phases of implementation, the master trainers had the capability to provide all the training and consulting services initially supplied by the paid outside consultants. Since TQI is an ongoing rather than a "one-shot" process, the ultimate goal for VHA's implementation was to develop local trainers with sufficient consulting skills to keep the TQI cultural change alive and well. As the pilot sites' training capabilities increased, the master trainers would be available to assist those facilities that still needed outside help and then begin to take on other training duties within VHA.

The initial phase of the implementation began in August 1991.

During this part of the cycle, VHA relied entirely on paid consultants for training and consulting services at the thirteen Phase I sites. The second phase began in June 1992. During this part of the implementation, VHA relied upon a combination of RMEC trainers and paid consultants for the continuing training needs of the Phase I sites, while the paid consultants moved on to bring another twenty-five sites into total quality. Those sites were also used for the "on-site" training of the master trainers developed during the first phase. The cost in consulting fees for each of these two phases was approximately the same. However, with a greater reliance upon the use of master trainers to provide ever-increasing portions of the training, the number of paid consultant days per facility was reduced (the total remained roughly the same because the number of facilities doubled in Phase II). Training for the remaining 140 VA medical centers, where primary reliance for training and consultative services was upon the master trainers, was expected to be accomplished with far less cost than that required for Phases I and II. The elimination of the routine use of paid consultants would significantly reduce the cost of bringing each VA hospital into the total quality culture, enabling VHA to bring the remaining 140 sites on board at a fraction of the cost of the original thirteen. If problems arose, the paid consultants could still be called in. Use of VHA's own trainers and consultants would be much more cost-effective than paying over $1600 per day to outside consultants, and the locally trained VHA staff members that were recruited by the executive assistants for TQI to assist with training at the facility level would be the most cost-effective of all.

At the end of fiscal year 1992, a period that encompassed Phase I of the implementation, VHA had expended only slightly more than $157,000 (not including VHA salary costs) and had obtained more than three hundred training sessions for the master trainers. A little more than a third of these sessions, 114, occurred at central locations and were taught by an external consultant. The remaining two-thirds of the training episodes took place in the various hospitals, where the master trainers either were actively trained by consultants, who were themselves involved in training the local hospital staff, or actually did some of the training themselves, while a consultant observed and mentored the process. Additional funds were spent that year on educating the executive assistants for TQI and for other costs, such as travel expenses for physician consultants. Visits by VHA physician consultants to the pilot sites were not considered formal education sessions, although often a certain amount of teaching went on between the consultant and the hospital's staff physicians.

Information reported to the St. Louis continuing education center from the Phase I hospitals during fiscal year 1992 also tracked the training activity at each of the individual facilities. By the end of the year, the master trainers reported that the multiple training sessions at each hospital had provided a total of 9,680 employees with awareness training. At the Lexington VA hospital, a two-hour presentation on awareness, presented twenty-two times over a two-week period, succeeded in covering all 1,100 employees in the hospital! The Columbus, Ohio, outpatient clinic used a one-and-a-half- to two-hour presentation, presented six times in a brief period, and also covered all of their employees. Not everyone used the mass inoculation approach, but those who did contributed heavily to the numbers of VHA employees who were exposed to the concepts of TQI early in their hospital's journey.

In addition to the nearly ten thousand employees given basic awareness training, 472 employees received specific training in the concepts of team leadership or team facilitation. A total of 1,199 employees were trained in the roles and responsibilities of team members during this same time. Even before the first year of the implementation effort was over, VHA had successfully laid a solid foundation of training that reached a large number of employees. Furthermore, the training methodology—which stressed the concomitant training of VHA's own master trainers—was further shifting the cost of training from the expensive use of consultants to the more appropriate use of internal experts.

In fiscal year 1993 the training continued through Phase II, embracing a total of thirty-eight hospitals. In most of these facilities, the training schedules were similar. Awareness training came first, emphasizing either the entire workforce or particular groups of involved employees, such as upper management, key members of steering committees, and the members of early implementation teams. Next came training in assessment methods and the functions of team members, leaders, and facilitators. A few hospitals tried to provide training on very specific topics, such as the use of

TQI tools, to a broad spectrum of employees early in the implementation phase, but most were so busy with other training efforts that they were content to follow VHA's recommendations that such training be made available to teams on a "just-in-time" (JIT) basis when their work required it.

Some facilities used a technique of concentrated training for a manageable few early in the process, with the intent of keeping the implementation moving along based on the activity and effectiveness of these trained employees. One example of this kind of plan existed at the Jackson, Mississippi, VA hospital. The leadership, the consultant, and the master trainer devised a schedule of two and a half days for training the members of six teams. Two teams were trained at a time, and a special four-day facilitator course was offered to about thirty interested employees. At the conclusion of this aggressive training period, the hospital found itself with the capacity to charter several teams to address high-priority items and to support those teams with well-trained members and facilitators right from the beginning.

One of the Phase II sites, the domiciliary at White City, Oregon, was particularly interested in getting a wide spectrum of employees trained and involved in the TQI process as soon as possible. Top management and key leaders at the White City facility had been involved and pursuing training for their employees even before the national program began. They had contracted with the Juran Institute in July 1991 to provide sixteen hours of training in awareness and team member responsibilities to 150 of their key managers; this impressive beginning continued, with ongoing dedication to the need for specific training for their whole workforce. To meet these ambitious goals, the leadership at White City developed and met some specific objectives, such as developing an experienced cadre of team leaders and facilitators with knowledge and experience in using advanced tools and techniques, maintaining an internal capability to provide whatever training was needed, and seeing that JIT training was provided to active teams as needed throughout their period of activity. The thoroughness of the White City approach is illustrated in Table 11.1, which depicts the broad spectrum of training the facility offered and the degree to which it penetrated the workforce.

At White City, through the diligence and perseverance of top

**Table 11.1. Training Spectrum and Penetration
at the White City Domiciliary.**

Training Type	Description	Number Eligible	Number Attended	Percentage
Awareness	4–8 hours	359	330	92%
Team member	16 hours	359	261	73%
Leader/facilitator	16 hours	17	17	100%
Customer satisfaction	8 hours	359	101	28%
Deployment	16 hours	54	54	100%
Organizational culture	8 hours	73	73	100%
Council	16 hours	4	4	100%

Awareness: Brief overview of TQI

Team member: Explanation of roles

Leader/facilitator: Training for team leaders or facilitators

Customer satisfaction: Training for employees in customer service and satisfaction

Deployment: Training in using assessment and chartering concepts at the departmental level

Organizational culture: Training for managers in facilitating change in employee expectations and behavior

Council: Training for steering council members, all facets presented

management, virtually every employee was exposed to training covering a variety of TQI concepts and tools. The facility had received more than ten thousand hours of training by mid-1995; this equates to an average of twenty-seven hours per employee of specific, targeted training in support of the facility's TQI efforts, supplied entirely by internal facility staff. Training from the outside master trainers was in addition to this amount. Clearly the advantage to the White City facility's approach lies in the ability to have so many employees actively and productively engaged in so many process improvement teams.

Furthering its move to decentralize the training process, VHA encouraged individual hospitals to develop their own local training corps. The executive assistants for TQI at different hospitals used a variety of strategies to select assistant trainers as well as apprentice leaders and facilitators. Some opted for local personnel who were already involved in training of different types. At the San Diego VA hospital, a conscious effort was made to select mid-level managers to become in-house trainers and facilitators for cross-functional and department-level teams. This enabled these middle managers to learn the new skills they needed to work with their own staff as well as to promote quality improvement within their own portions of the organization. Much of the success of the TQI implementation rested upon how well trained these middle managers were (see Chapter Ten).

In order to develop internal expertise across the entire VHA system, the executive assistants for TQI needed to have some knowledge of local staff interests and skills, and they had to seek out staff with knowledge of TQI philosophy and concepts who were willing to participate. The material presented in the various training sessions was not complex or difficult (with the exception of the more advanced statistical tools). Therefore it was more important early on to find enthusiastic supporters of the total quality philosophy who were good communicators than it was to find good technicians or people with an in-depth knowledge of the TQI process. But when the time came to get into the more advanced and esoteric statistical methodologies, it was better to have some local staff with such expertise available to consult with the team. Research and psychology services at VA hospitals were good sources for such experts. Psychology staff were an important resource to teams developing questionnaires or surveys and needing assistance in norming processes. The San Diego hospital even put together a measurement team to provide training and assistance in measurement and analysis to any team that needed it.

The methods for selecting employees to be trained as team leaders was marked by philosophical differences of opinion between certain consultants and some of the executive assistants for TQI. The conventional wisdom for selection of team leaders was to choose individuals that were knowledgeable of the process under study. The executive assistants for TQI often found, however, that people with good leadership skills, even if they were not knowledgeable about the process under evaluation, could provide excellent leadership for teams. The fact was that the "right" leader from an organizational perspective was not always the proper choice from a human viewpoint. Therefore, staff selected for training as team leaders were chosen either because of their knowledge of the process under assessment or because of their proved leadership skills. As the quality culture becomes ingrained in the organization, VHA will find it more common for natural team leaders to come from those who know and work with the process under study. But for the pilot effort it was important that team leaders and facilitators be drawn from the pool of informal leaders in each facility, to enhance the likelihood of their, and the organization's, success.

Throughout fiscal year 1993, the continuing education center in St. Louis continued to track the training provided by consultants to the cadre of master trainers. Increasingly the training was taking place at the various hospitals, as the master trainers became more involved and responsible for the bulk of the training at each institution. In fiscal year 1993 there were 120 sessions of training for master trainers by consultants at a central location (away from the hospital setting and involving more didactic presentations); this number is not much different from the 114 such episodes provided in fiscal year 1992. However, in 1993 there were 378 training sessions at the individual VA hospitals; in fiscal year 1992 there were only 169 such sessions. The shift of the major responsibility for training from the consultants to the master trainers can be easily tracked by the level of master trainer involvement in training at each hospital. Each of the on-site sessions represented training not only for hospital staff but also for the master trainer, under the tutelage of the outside consultant. During fiscal year 1993, VHA spent some $414,776 on a total of 618 such on-site sessions. In addition to those sessions mentioned above, there was training for master trainers in advanced skills (53 sessions), 45 visits from physician advisors, and 22 sessions of miscellaneous training for executive assistants and master trainers. The average cost of travel for each session, whether on-site or centrally located, was $671—a real bargain in any circumstance.

Problems and Experiences

As with any TQI implementation, the importance of the role of the leadership—in this case, the hospital directors and chiefs of staff—

cannot be overemphasized. Sahney and Warden (1991) assert that TQI simply will not work in organizations where the support and commitment from top management is not solid. Although VHA's experience in this regard was not substantially different from that seen in other settings—both health care and industrial—the examples it offers are useful and revealing. Repeatedly, the consultants and master trainers reported that the implementation was affected by the attitude and involvement of the hospital director in ways that were at times almost palpable. One example comes from the Albany VA hospital, where the director was unable to attend a morning session of awareness training. After some of the concerns and murmurings about the importance of such training were reported to him, the director appeared for the afternoon session, took off his coat, rolled up his sleeves, and became a part of the proceedings. At least one of the physicians present at that session said, "Well, if the director is here, this must be important."

At the Lexington VA hospital, the director and most members of the quality leadership team (QLT) were personally present for twenty of the twenty-two training sessions stressing awareness. Not only were these key players there, they spoke to the employees and endorsed their activity and time expenditure on the process. They remained available for a question-and-answer period and further cemented in the minds of the employees that they believed this effort to be worthwhile. Similarly, the director at the Dayton VA hospital attended and made opening comments at virtually every one of the training sessions. In addition, Dayton's QLT met with every process improvement team immediately after their training and chartering; this provided an excellent opportunity for both to understand each other's role, their charter, and the support they could expect during their activity. In these facilities the mood was clearly upbeat; the positive influence of leadership involvement was evident. Unfortunately, this was not the case in every facility.

During Phase I and Phase II, there was turnover in the directorship of twelve facilities—nearly a third of the pilot sites. The shifting priorities and general uncertainty that accompanied such major changes in top management were undeniable negatives in the VHA experience. The Columbus outpatient clinic experienced such a change in directorship; during the interregnum, one of the major department heads sat in the rear of the room and read the newspaper during a QLT training session. This individual obviously believed that TQI was not a major interest of top management. At the Las Vegas outpatient clinic, the initial phases of training and implementation went smoothly and had the thorough and active endorsement of both the director and the chief of staff. The first two teams in the facility received sixteen to thirty-two hours of training and effectively brought in their improvements (including reductions in cycle time and increases in patient satisfaction). Then the facility hit a brick wall: other priorities—including a major construction project and the negotiation of a unique sharing agreement with the U.S. Air Force—intervened. Then the director was reassigned, and the process stalled. Most of the planned training was postponed and later canceled in the face of the difficulties in handling these internal issues.

As noted elsewhere, published information on the attitudes and beliefs of VA hospital directors (Tindill, Al-Assaf, & Gentling, 1993, pp. 45–52) indicates their understanding of the critical need for their support and personal involvement in the TQI process. Apparently, they also believe that TQI will actually improve the quality of care at their facility, so the question of motivation for making the personal investment is less uncertain. The survey also noted that the directors expected results within the first year; it was less certain in their minds that TQI would decrease total health care costs, however, so exactly what results they expected was not clear. In view of these findings and the generally positive support the TQI implementation received from almost every sitting director, the slowed progress during and immediately following a change in director likely resulted from uncertainty in the facility about the new director's priorities.

As noted earlier, sometimes facilities need to create special support functions to assist their teams and employees at certain times. The measurement team created at the San Diego VA hospital is one such example. Another is the trainer and facilitator support group put together at the Lexington VA hospital in response to the stress placed on trainers by high-speed awareness training and the increasing number of active teams. This group was originally conceived of as a straightforward support group, but their focus and activity changed quite early in their history. They found that one important support activity was to keep track of the various training activities going on throughout the hospital and bring some degree of coordination to the process. Quite soon they found themselves taking control of the training schedule for the hospital—to the delight of the QLT—and lessening the confusion and pressure that led to the formation of the group to begin with.

There were wide variations in the number of trainers needed at each facility. Some of the larger facilities, like the complex Brooklyn VA hospital, had as many as sixty trainers to meet the needs of their teams. Other, smaller facilities could get along with only two or three trainers. While size is an obvious factor in determining the number of in-house trainers needed, the level of activity may actually be more important. The speed with which the TQI process could be deployed in a given hospital was more often dependent on the availability of sufficient trainers to handle its particular training needs (such as training in team dynamics, assessment, basic awareness, team leader roles, and so on). Often, plans to charter more improvement teams and put them to work were impeded by the lack of time to train new trainers, because all available trainers were supporting active groups. Occasionally, success itself, and the resultant higher expectations, created unreasonable demands. Further, the trainers became steadily more aware that they needed additional training in the next level of information, just to remain current as well as to be able to bring new concepts to the table with the teams they were to support. As one of the master trainers put it, "training is forever."

Evaluation

The use of indicators and measures to assess processes is always emphasized in TQI, and the training process is no exception. It is important to identify key indicators to use in monitoring the effectiveness of training. As the executive assistant for TQI from Chicago's West Side hospital stated, "The best measures of effectiveness are the opportunities for improvement identified, recommendations made, and process improvements implemented." However, measuring training effectiveness by focusing on process indicators may leave unanswered the question "Does it work to improve care or reduce costs?" Training may enable staff to efficiently assess a process, collect the necessary data for analyzing it, and even make substantive changes in it. But if these changes cannot be directly tied to improvements in the quality of care or to reductions in the cost of delivering it, there is significant risk of losing the backing and involvement of both management and the clinical staff.

For most of the Phase I and II facilities, evaluation of the TQI implementation involved more process measurement than outcome assessment. The number of employees trained, as an indicator of the penetration of training into the workforce, was a major point of emphasis. Likewise, a high number of teams chartered, supported, and bringing on change was considered evidence of progress and success in the implementation. While these measures do indicate the level of involvement and the degree of TQI activity at a hospital, there is a need for more focused outcome measures. Many of the teams were able to show improvements in the processes they addressed, such as a reduction in waiting times in certain clinics and an increase in chart availability for outpatient visits. While this evidence of success from TQI activity was available at the local level, no attempt was made to report these measurements to any centralized office. Thus there is no database from which to draw conclusive evidence that the process worked in each hospital or that the outcome of TQI involvement was a demonstrable improvement in health care quality. What was available for review in judging the success of the pilot phase were process measures and anecdotal reports from the master trainers, who had visited the individual sites and worked closely with employees from top management to the most junior members of the workforce.

One of the master trainers, Marisa Palkuti, noted that often there were no set measures to determine the effectiveness of training, although trained teams commonly expressed the belief that they were able to achieve their goals much more quickly than they would have had they not been trained in TQI. Palkuti also noted, "The 'outcomes' of training, particularly substantial changes in the way people work, may be more determined by organizational barriers within the hospital than by the training itself." This is particularly true when mid-level managers are not actively brought into the training or team process; their downstream lack of enthusiasm or involvement—or outright obstruction—may cause the process to fail, even when high-quality training has been presented to and learned by the rest of the employees.

In that same vein, Karen McCoy, another of the master trainers, noted that she did not see many teams or hospitals establishing measures of effectiveness for training at the beginning of their involvement. She further noted that such measures would have to be focused on some form of outcome related to the process under scrutiny: "This kind of training doesn't show effectiveness unless it is tied to action or performance. This is not skills training." Even a measure of team activity in the form of data and analysis must be handled with some caution. For example, one team produced a professional-looking bar graph of the "reasons" the care process they were evaluating was not working well. On close questioning, however, it was revealed that the "reasons" were actually a list of opinions from a variety of people about why they thought the care process didn't work, not a data-driven analysis of actual measurements. This anecdote underscores the need for outcome measures (and the story itself is a measure of the understanding the team members had about measurement after their training).

There is no widely accepted measure of effectiveness for some kinds of training, such as awareness training. Sometimes the only "measure" of success or failure was the consultant's or master trainer's impressions concerning whether a certain form of training had been effective at a particular hospital. Here, too, the role played and support given by the hospital director and chief of staff seemed to make a real impression on the employees and outside reviewers. One of the master trainers said such kinds of training represented "a lot of money down a rat hole" if the director and other members of top management were not visibly present and actively supportive of the training and the philosophy it represented. For those hospitals where the director and chief of staff were involved and supportive, the penetration of the training was greater, the number of initial teams chartered was higher, and the impression from the employees and master trainers was that the training had been more effective than in those facilities where top management's role was less visible.

For the evaluation of teams, the executive assistant for TQI, the process owner, even the team members themselves must accept the responsibility to monitor progress and, ultimately, the effectiveness of their efforts. The decision about what success will look like should be made at the time the team is chartered. When it appears a team is experiencing difficulty in meeting its predetermined milestones, a consultant, either internal or external, should meet with the team to assess the difficulty and determine if additional training is needed. In addition, the executive assistant for TQI should measure the results being achieved against the anticipated results to determine if the activity is on track. Teams must not be permitted to flounder about without receiving assistance, guidance, or additional training if necessary. It does not take long for team members to lose interest and stop coming to the meetings if progress is not steady. For these reasons, the number of teams that fail to produce meaningful outcomes and improvements may be one measure of the effectiveness of training as well as the adequacy of follow-up on team activities. Eventually, monitoring and continuously improving the process—including setting and measuring outcomes—must become the responsibility of the process owner. (This is, in fact, the essence of the TQI philosophy.) Continual measurement of processes by quality assurance personnel at the facility takes away the primary responsibility of the process owner right from the start, and it should not become a way of doing business in a TQI environment.

Sustaining

As noted above, "training is forever." This might be interpreted by some as "Once trained, always trained," but in a TQI environment it means that the need for training continues as long as employees are moving forward on their TQI journey. New employees need training, some employees need retraining, and many employees want additional training as they become more involved and see the need for more personal skills and knowledge. VHA's experience at its Phase I and II pilot sites revealed a spectrum of needs, causes for those needs, and different ways to meet them.

The assessments of the master trainers allowed us to see very clearly that the thirty-eight hospitals in the two phases were at different levels of knowledge and expertise at all times. This was not simply due to the time difference between their starting dates. The attitudes and prior involvement of the staff and the director played a major role as well, as did a variety of local issues, including personalities. Turnover in the director's office was obviously a negative influence. Other factors included poorly defined issues such as the scheduling of training, the energy of the employees, and the existence of other external pressures (such as an impending Joint Commission on Accreditation of Healthcare Organizations survey).

Lessons Learned

The three most important concepts learned in VHA about sustaining the TQI philosophy were as follows:

- Keeping local trainers fresh, eager, and involved.
- Continually provide new challenges and training for employees.
- Work the TQI philosophy into the day-to-day activities of the entire workforce, rather than just stressing them in team settings and when looking for improvements in nonfunctional processes.

Several of the facilities noted the need for more training and more local trainers as their activity increased and more teams were chartered. The usual solution to such increased demand was to draw upon tested employees. Some individuals went from one team to another without any break in the level of their involvement. With only a few trained leaders or facilitators in a hospital, the load may quickly become more than they can handle. Obviously, the answer is to train more employees in the roles and responsibilities of team members, leaders, and facilitators, but this is not always easily accomplished when the local trainers are also busy keeping up with training and their own work load. The important lesson is to always be providing training for employees, in several categories: new employees should be trained in awareness, those not requiring further training in awareness should be introduced to assessment and team functions, those who have had team member training should be exposed to leadership and facilitator training, and so on.

Overly aggressive training schedules must be avoided, however. Not only does the massive training time required for such an endeavor pull away needed talent from active teams, it also raises an expectation in the workforce that is difficult to meet in a timely fashion. There must be a delicate balance between the number of trained individuals and the activity level in the hospital. Early on it is probably best to proceed at a steady pace, simply matching training needs to the needs of the original teams. As their needs grow, however, the demand for training may increase exponentially. Not only is there a linear increase in demand paralleling the number of new teams chartered, there is also a need to provide the next level of training to many of the employees who were among the first to be trained. At that point these individuals will be ready to begin assuming the role of trainer for such topics as tools training, statistical analysis, and so on, and they will have to be trained in these skills. Furthermore, the effective trainers will have been hard at work for some time and will need to be relieved of such intense involvement for a while—but there may be no one to take their place.

Many facilities and executive assistants for TQI learned the need to strike a fine balance with trainers and their assignments. Asking them to train too frequently could overburden them unfairly and lead to burnout. Across the pilot sites, many good trainers were lost in this fashion. At the same time, trainers need to use their training skills; they need to teach the course material frequently enough to retain mastery over the material. Good trainers enjoy the classroom interaction involved in participatory training. However, such interactive training can be tiring. To remain productive, these sessions need to be spaced out a little. As one trainer from Dallas observed, "Too little time between training sessions leaves me exhausted physically, mentally, and emotionally. I tend to get 'flat' as a presenter, and my teaching suffers as a result." The proper spacing, like so much else in training, varies from person to person and must be arranged individually between the trainer and the executive assistant.

Sustaining the training effort became a problem in some facilities as trainers burned out, became involved in other responsibilities, or left the facility. In addition, interludes developed in which no training was required, as trained teams did their work or resources were shifted to deal with elements of change coming from a variety of other sources. Changes in leadership, especially at the executive level, before the facility culture had changed often hampered the deployment of such change, thereby reducing the demand for training. Executive assistants were then faced with having to find and train new trainers, or reenergize the existing ones.

In addition to difficulties in sustaining the training effort, some of the executive assistants for TQI found that the implementation plan did not incorporate or emphasize the need to reinforce training, except during the time employees were actually assigned to work on a team. As Karl Albrecht (1988) points out, "One of the worst misuses of training as an organizational resource is simply training people with no follow-through. . . . Training, all by itself, accomplishes relatively little. It can give people new ideas, new skills, and new attitudes. But it is not the primary determinant of the way they behave on the job. What determines how they behave on the job is the leadership they receive from their supervisors and the reinforcement signals they get from their work environment" (pp. 188–189). Ideally, trained team members begin using process analysis in everything they do once they learn how to use the tools. But this requires the strong support of supervisors willing to provide them with the additional resources they need to actually use what they have learned. This (previously unidentified) need became a major hurdle for the successful implementation of TQI in the pilot sites; the most successful sites were those best able to balance facility needs with individual employees' needs. An example is the San Diego VA hospital; early on they identified and trained over twenty employees to be facilitators, and they kept them busy with a variety of activities, ranging from retreat management to team-based data analysis, without overburdening any of them.

Two ways to maintain the interest and capability of trainers are to provide them with the new training they need and to allow them to use the skills they have gained in activities that are more time-efficient than one-on-one training. Team teaching will accomplish the latter, but it may be a new experience for many trainers. Those who tried it at the pilot sites discovered some very real advantages to the concept. First, team teaching enables them to get assistance from their colleague sitting in the back of the room. For example, sometimes instructors have difficulty understanding a question from someone on the team, or they don't really provide a complete answer. The instructor sitting in the back of the room can often perceive this difficulty and add additional comments to clarify a response. Team teachers must feel comfortable enough with each other to allow that kind of interchange. Second, in a hospital emergencies do occur, and if one of the instructors needs to leave, the other can still teach the class without the disruption of having to abandon the activity because of the crisis. Third, when a class will be breaking into smaller work groups, two instructors can provide better attention to the different groups, to ensure that they are on target with whatever task is assigned. Finally, team teaching is not nearly as exhausting as teaching alone, because time is available to sit down, review some notes for the next section, or just drink some coffee and not be on stage all the time.

For the employees, the purpose of training and working with teams is not simply to "fix" the problems identified by the assessment. Unfortunately, many employees believe TQI is primarily used to fix problems; although TQI concepts are useful for fixing problems, this represents a relatively low level of sophistication in the use of TQI tools and philosophy. A more mature and responsible use of the continuous improvement concept is to prevent problems before they occur. This requires forward thinking on the part of process owners and designers and the application of the TQI philosophy in their day-to-day work. Simply put, for the prevention aspect of continuous improvement to be manifest at a given hospital, the entire workforce must incorporate the concepts and tools of TQI into their daily routine; the culture would have to change from top-down direction to self-managed activities. This type of activity would indicate, in the most compelling manner possible, that the training in TQI and the implementation of the continuous improvement philosophy had been effective. There are a few such instances developing across the VHA system, and they deserve notice.

At the Hines VA hospital, where John Fears started the leadership down the TQI path in the late 1980s, the boiler plant crew had some experience with TQI flowcharting and recognized the power of the tool for helping them analyze their plant operation. They obtained some computer software with flowcharting capability and began to use it to analyze their own daily activities. They charted their processes and identified several areas in which they could streamline their own activities. As a result of their continued attention to the use of this one tool, the boiler plant at Hines is strikingly more efficient and the employees feel they are making a difference in the overall capability of Hines to deliver cost-effective, high-quality health care.

At the White City domiciliary, one of the incentive work therapy activities is the construction of pizza paddles for handling pizza pies in high-heat ovens. These paddles are constructed from blocks of mountain ash that are glued cross-grain to enhance their strength and then planed to size before being shipped to retailers for sale. The entire process takes more than forty individual steps, from warehousing the unglued blocks to packaging the final paddles for shipping. Employees and patients involved in the incentive work therapy program at White City produced a flowchart of the process and actively collected data at nearly every point to continually monitor their accuracy and identify problems and areas that needed attention and improvement. This same kind of attention to process detail is beginning to be evident in the facility's treatment processes as well; one example is the recent reduction of the intake processing time for new patients in the alcohol and drug treatment program from eleven days to two days. Across the system, the use of TQI methods in the everyday work of employees is beginning to make itself evident.

In May 1995, VHA held a national conference for executive assistants and quality managers in Atlanta. Over the course of several days, these heavily involved local experts exchanged concepts and ideas and presented information in poster sessions, concurrent sessions, and plenary sessions. Before this conference, they were asked to complete a survey detailing some of their activities. Detailed answers were submitted by 67 facilities; extrapolating those answers to the entire system of 172 hospitals yielded some interesting information about the level of activity and productivity across the broad face of VHA. If the extrapolation can be accepted, by mid-1995 VHA had provided training to

110,700 employees in awareness

20,340 employees in team member roles

4140 employees in team facilitation skills

5940 employees in team leadership

234 employees in the application of Baldrige criteria to VHA settings

Furthermore, the extrapolation indicates that 1,152 process improvement teams had probably been chartered across the system and had completed their work; another 1,350 such teams were still in progress and actively pursuing improvement at that time. In addition, the facilities reported data that indicated over 160 clinical pathways had been completed and about 270 more were in active development. It was obvious at that point that the emphasis on developing internal expertise and capability for training in TQI concepts and tools had been a major success and that VHA was clearly gaining momentum and experience daily.

References

Albrecht, K. (1988). *At America's service: How corporations can revolutionize the way they treat their customers.* Homewood, IL: Dow Jones-Irwin.

Ernst & Young Quality Improvement Consulting Group. (1990). *Total quality: An executive's guide for the 1990s.* Homewood, IL: Irwin/Apics.

Gitlow, H. S., & Gitlow, S. J. (1987). *The Deming guide to quality and competitive position.* Englewood Cliffs, NJ: Prentice-Hall.

Sahney, V. K., & Warden, G. (1991). The quest for quality and productivity in health services. *Frontiers of Health Services Management, 7*(4), 2–40, 55–66.

Tindill, B. S., Al-Assaf, A. F., & Gentling, S. J. (1993). Total quality improvement: A study of Veterans Affairs medical center directors and QA coordinators. *American Journal of Medical Quality, 8,* 45–52.

Vogt, J. F., & Murrell, K. L. (1990). *Empowerment in organizations.* San Diego, CA: Pfeiffer.

Part Four

Outcomes

Chapter Twelve

Early Experiences: Some Firsthand Accounts

Edited by M. Jo MacDonald and Gene D. Mickelson

This chapter presents fifteen vignettes describing total quality improvement (TQI) team activity in VA hospitals. These vignettes describe actual solutions to actual problems encountered by TQI practitioners in Phase I and II sites. While not a random statistical sampling, they constitute a fair representation of the kinds of issues the early teams addressed. The examples provided are reflective of countless other stories from across the VA health care system that can be found among the over six hundred team descriptions in VHA's centralized TQI teams database. The database is managed by VHA's Quality Management Institute, located in Durham, North Carolina. Input to the database is made by TQI practitioners throughout the health care system. This database is a ready reference, describing what kinds of teams exist throughout the VA health care system and listing key team members who can be contacted for information about their team. Another source of information on team activity is VHA's performance excellence database, which focuses on describing team activities and accomplishments, applications for the Robert W. Carey Quality Award, and the VHA publication *Sharing Innovations Among VA Clinicians*.

The vignettes described in this chapter focus mainly on early TQI process action teams in Phase I and Phase II facilities. It should be noted that acronyms and terminology may vary among sites, reflecting the diversity among VHA facilities. A good example of diversity is seen in the titles of the leadership groups responsible for chartering and monitoring TQI teams: quality leadership team (QLT), quality council, TQI leadership team, quality executive board, and TQI steering committee. While the leadership groups may have different names, they all share common attributes: these groups direct the TQI efforts in VA hospitals, and the majority of the members generally come from the ranks of senior and mid-level managers.

These vignettes clearly show the evolving presence of a TQI structure in the VA health care system. As noted earlier, an early intent of the framers of VHA's TQI plan was to implement a *system* of TQI. To this end, they intended that certain core TQI practices be installed systemwide; these practices are clearly evident in these early descriptions of TQI teams. Most teams, for example, operated under the auspices of a governing *council* or *committee*. Most teams received a *charter* from that body to solve a problem, and that charter emanated from some kind of *assessment*. Teams were provided with *leaders* and *facilitators* and received *training* in TQI principles and techniques. They used a variety of *tools* to analyze often complex issues and generally followed some version of a *plan, do, check, act* process. All of these structures and processes are evidence of a TQI system evolving in VHA.

The topics selected for the early teams mirrored the diversity of the issues they faced. The majority of the teams concentrated on administrative processes, but many of those processes had direct implications on patient care. Clearly, the front entrance congestion at San Antonio, the employee training program at Jackson, access to policy and procedures at New York, and the decentralized hospital computer program (DHCP) document retrieval system at White City are administrative issues. Bed cleaning at Temple, the Drugs 'R' Us program at Dayton, and the medical records system at Reno and Albuquerque are also basically administrative processes, but they have clear patient care implications. On the other hand, the admissions process at Dallas, the patient assessment process at Minneapolis, and the outpatient timeliness policy at Big Spring and Lexington are essentially patient care issues that involve administrative processes. Finally, the total hip replacement, pneumovax, and transporting of critically ill patients processes at Albany, Portland, and Loma Linda, respectively, are purely patient-focused issues.

The stories are told by actual practitioners who were involved in the team activity. Each story is introduced by italicized editors' comments highlighting select aspects of the team process.

Administrative Processes

Front Entrance Congestion Team

This story illustrates a basic fact of "TQI life"; namely, teams often can solve problems that have defied individual or piecemeal efforts for years. Chronic problems are often good targets for TQI intervention—teams can be powerful tools. More importantly, this story illustrates graphically the importance of one of the fundamental pillars of TQI—focus on the customer. In this case, many of the customers who were creating a problem for the hospital were enlisted in the improvement process.

Congestion at the front entrance to the Audie L. Murphy Memorial Veterans Hospital in San Antonio had been a chronic problem over a number of years, defying resolution in spite of management's best efforts through policing and signage. Patients, visitors, and employees coming into the building early in the morning were met by individuals who congregated at a seating area just outside the front entrance. This crowd was characterized by many smokers, loud music, inappropriate comments, whistling, and "cat calling." San Antonio was the first hospital in the VA system to adopt a nonsmoking policy, in 1988. The front entrance congestion was an unintended byproduct of that policy, because many patients used the area to smoke outside the hospital. Congestion at the front entrance increased during the day, reaching a particularly offensive level around 4:30 P.M. Departing employees, particularly women, were the targets of stares, comments, and sometimes intimidating behavior.

By mid-1993, during the assessment phase of VHA's TQI implementation, a team of hospital employees had set about to learn from patients, patients' families, volunteers, employees, and other groups their perception of the many services provided by the facility. Offensive conditions at the front entrance were identified as a major issue people were concerned about. The safety committee had also identified this issue as a high priority. One employee had tripped over the curb trying to avoid verbal harassment, fallen, and injured her ankle. There were reports of employees almost being hit by automobiles as they exited the crowded sidewalk. Complaint mail continued to flow in regularly to the director's office about this situation.

During this period, the quality executive board (QEB) was creating the necessary infrastructure for TQI deployment, consisting of training, awards and recognition, measurement, quality assurance–TQI integration, and service-level quality deployment. The QEB chartered and deployed teams in four areas: operating room start-up times, outpatient clinic no-shows, eye clinic management practices, and front entrance congestion.

The congestion team was headed by the chief quality management officer, who was also the TQI executive assistant. The facilitator was Gloria Sloan, associate chief of the nursing service, who added the perspective of psychiatry to the team. Other members included a representative from the Veterans of Foreign Wars service organization; the chief of medical center police and security; a public relations specialist; the chief of the volunteer service; an electrician from the engineering service, who represented the local American Federation of Government Employees union; and the assistant chief of the engineering service.

The team received two days of team training conducted by a consultant and a regional medical education center (RMEC) TQI master trainer, and they set about the task of reviewing the problems and recommending improvements at the front entrance. Early on, the team recognized that the needs of those congregated in the front entrance had to be understood and met. Early in its work, the team used a cause-and-effect diagram as a brainstorming tool to help in identifying the many possible causes of the congestion problem. The results were used to develop focused interview protocols, which were completed with fifty individuals in the area to begin to understand who the users were and why they were there. Figure 12.1 shows the data received from the interviews.

These data show that the majority (over 60 percent) were there to smoke. Other data showed that most were patients. By understanding the needs of the people who were causing the congestion—the patients, visitors, those awaiting transportation, and employees—and by focusing on why they were there, the team was able to design alternatives that would address their needs and resolve the congestion.

Figure 12.1. Reasons for Being in the Front Entrance Area.

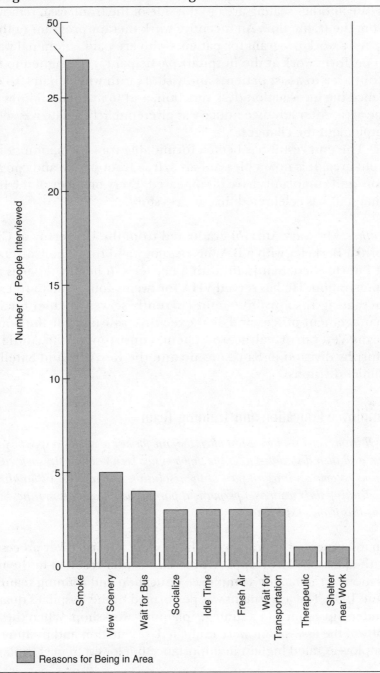

Reasons for Being in Area

Recommendations were made to remove existing benches and create another seating area to the side of the front area, removed from the traffic flow. An incentive work therapy program (a therapeutic work program for patients who are paid a nominal wage to perform work at the hospital) participant was assigned to the front area to assist patients and visitors with wheelchairs, to enhance the information desk function, and to maintain tidiness in the area. After advance notice was given publicly, a date was set to implement the changes.

The end result has been a formidable transformation of the front area. It is now a pleasant area, free from smoke and congestion, and complaints have disappeared. Every member of the hospital staff has celebrated this success story.

Author: Mr. Gary Anziani graduated from the University of California, Berkeley with a B.A. in sociology and from the University of Puerto Rico, San Juan, with a master's in health services administration. He has served VHA for twenty-four years in roles of increasing responsibility and currently serves as chief quality management officer and TQI executive assistant for the South Texas Veterans Healthcare System, consisting of the Audie L. Murphy division in San Antonio and the Kerrville and Satellite Clinics divisions.

Employee Education and Training Team

TQI teams come and go. Most often they are formed to resolve a specific problem and then disbanded after the problem has been resolved. In some cases, teams become an integral part of the resolution and are institutionalized, continuing their work as a permanent part of their hospital's routine. Such was this team's experience.

An assessment of critical success factors and associated key processes at the Jackson, Mississippi, VA medical center resulted in the formation of the facility's employee education and training team in June 1993. The assessment was performed by the hospital's quality leadership council in a strategic planning workshop. When the results of the assessment were evaluated, orientation and training of employees rated highest in importance but lowest in performance of all the processes considered. Education and training was given priority over other major hospital processes that were identified as deficient, such as the admitting process, because the hospital had no comprehensive, organized training program and the staff were frustrated by their inability to get desired and needed training.

The education and training team was led by Richard J. Baltz, the hospital's associate director. The process improvement coordinator was the facilitator. Other members included the associate chief of staff for education, a nursing instructor, the chief of the library service, the clinical section chief of the food and nutrition service, and the quality manager. The mission of the team was to develop an organizational structure and process that would ensure comprehensive education and training for each employee. Specifically, the team was charged with identifying employee training needs, developing realistic approaches to training, developing a process to coordinate and document training, and addressing the new Joint Commission on Accreditation of Health Organizations' (JCAHO) standards on training.

Several members of the team had received previous process improvement training, so they were given just-in-time training by the facilitator. After preliminary discussion and development of the team's mission statement, the team set about identifying the components of an optimal training and education program, with a primary focus on the employee as the customer.

The team used flowcharting to assess the processes involved in the employee orientation and training process. Brainstorming techniques were used to determine what kinds of training resources were available, and these were displayed on a cause-and-effect diagram. Some of these data are shown in Figure 12.2. The team found many types of resources available for training; for example, RMEC classes and trainers, tuition support and reimbursement programs, and programs shared with the community.

The data collected illustrated several possible resources that could be developed into a coordinated and comprehensive education program. The current training program was examined in terms of the existing resources and processes devoted to training, and significant gaps were uncovered. The data in Figure 12.3 were derived from questionnaires completed by each discipline group and follow-up interviews conducted by one of the team members.

Figure 12.2. Impact of Training Resources on Creating a Coordinated, Comprehensive Education Program.

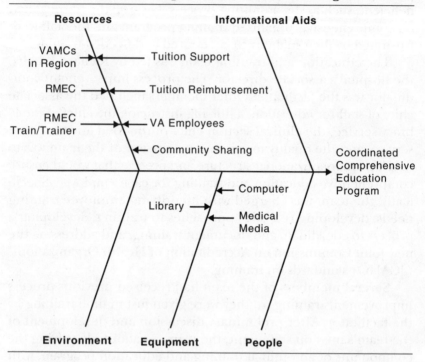

These data show the percent of hospital departments without key elements of a training program; namely, 40 percent lacked a formally documented orientation program for new employees, 70 percent did not have a written plan to address employee orientation and training, and over 80 percent had no written individual training plans.

All of these data were used by the team to develop recommendations for improving the overall quality of the education and training program. Based on the team's analysis, a plan that included recommendations for improvement was forwarded to the leadership council for review. The plan recommended several improvements:

Figure 12.3. Gaps in Employee Training.

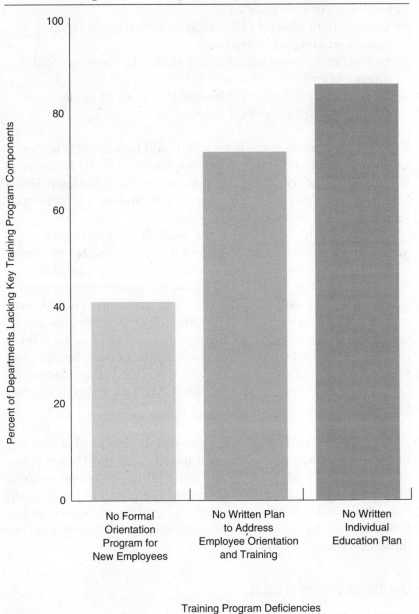

- A single education and training policy to integrate the existing patchwork of four policies
- A template to be used by hospital departments in creating department-level training plans
- An education committee, initially staffed by members of the education and training team
- An education specialist position in the office of the associate chief of staff for education

The council approved the team's plan and forwarded it to the senior leadership, who subsequently approved all of the recommendations. Once notice of this approval was received, the team, which now functioned as part of the education committee, began implementing the recommendations.

Because of this team's work, the facility's training program progressed from an ineffective, fragmented operation scattered among individual units to an effective, coordinated, comprehensive, facility-wide program. The hospital now has an integrated training and education program with offerings posted in weekly increments three to four weeks in advance. The postings tell employees what education and training sessions are scheduled in sufficient time for them to apply for needed courses. A major outcome of the education and training team's activity came in 1995, when the Jackson facility received extremely positive scores from JCAHO surveyors in all areas involving education and training.

Author: Carolyn C. Tindall is a registered dietitian with a master's degree in management. She graduated from the University of Southern Mississippi in 1979 and from Millsaps College in 1991. Carolyn has worked in the VHA health care system for thirteen years. Prior to becoming the process improvement coordinator at Jackson, she held the position of administrative section chief in the dietary service.

Document Retrieval Team

One of the drawbacks of TQI is the lament that it takes too long. TQI proponents answer this issue by pointing to the many positive outcomes for those who are willing to invest the time. This team took some time in its start-up phase, but they persevered and accomplished their goals. An interesting feature of this team's work, which undoubtedly contributed to its successful outcome, was the evaluation process for each meeting. Evaluations performed at each meeting were discussed at the next meeting.

The impetus for establishing the team described here came from an improvement opportunity in the information management and analysis section of the Malcolm Baldrige assessment. The team, based at the New York City VA medical center, was chartered specifically to improve access to medical center documents.

Team members were selected from a pool of volunteers and from services involved in accessing, disseminating, and/or aggregating medical center documents. Leading the team was Jack Davis, information resources management chief, and Leo Marinacci, public affairs officer, who served as the team facilitator. Prior to the team's first meeting, the leader and facilitator attended a four-hour workshop on team leadership and facilitation skills. At the conclusion of that workshop, a twelve-hour workshop on team-member skills was held for the entire team. The workshop focused on organizing the team to work efficiently and on basic process improvement tools and techniques.

In August 1992, the team began holding two-hour weekly meetings. It took several meetings for the team to decide on ground rules, meeting logistics, a mission statement, and a work plan. The mission statement that evolved was "to develop an efficient plan to improve upon the indexing, accessing, and circulation of Medical Center Letters, Medical Center Policy Memoranda, and Chief of Staff Memoranda." The team's work plan was based on a three-phased improvement process: (1) understand the current process, (2) gather and analyze customer and process data, and (3) select an area for improvement. In addition to developing a mission statement, the members decided to evaluate each team meeting using what they called a Team Wonderfulness Index, adapted from Peter R. Scholtes's index (1988). The index is a self-assessment tool completed by each member at the conclusion of each meeting. The team used a rating scale from 1 (best) to 5 (worst). The rating was based on members' perceptions of how well they had worked as a team at completing the meeting's objectives. Individual ratings were added and averaged to arrive at a team index rating for each meeting. While ratings varied, they were generally favorable, with the highest rating given to a team meeting attended by the medical center director. This is reflected in meeting 14 in Figure 12.4.

Through the use of flowcharts, fishbone diagrams, Pareto charts, brainstorming activities, and interviews of subject matter experts, the team acquired an extensive understanding of the document retrieval process and the needs and expectations of customers who used it. During the "long deliberations," as Davis called them,

Figure 12.4. Self-Assessments of Team Meetings.

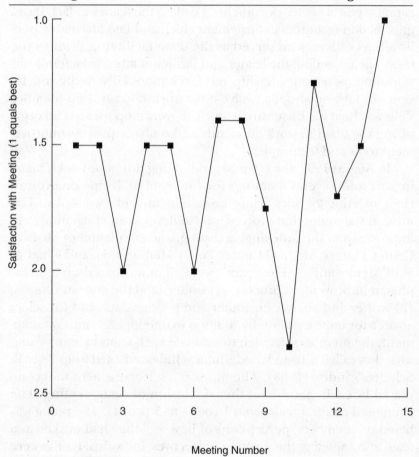

Meeting Number

the team "charted the entire process of generation, approval, indexing, and retrieval of the entire range of medical center documents, including medical center letters, policies, and chief of staff memoranda, as it existed. We took note of areas in which improvements could be made and gathered data to confirm or deny our assumptions." Customer satisfaction data was gathered through a poll of twenty-seven administrative and clinical services. The interview instrument was designed specifically to capture internal customers' perceptions of the current process and what they considered to be possible improvements. Survey responses, along with process data, were studied and used to design an automated program that accesses and retrieves medical center documents through the DHCP.

The result was a word processing system accessible to individuals who input, correct, and update medical center documents and to those who require access to read and/or print these documents. System features include a document directory and on-line help. Documents are encoded to include the document type, the service with primary responsibility, the date, a revision number, a subject heading, and a document list. Search capability exists by title for any given alphanumeric string (for example, the system will search for all documents with "A&MM" in the title) or by searching the text for key words (for example, the system will search for all documents with "bone scan'" in the text).

Twenty-eight clinical and administrative services are currently using the automated document retrieval system. Designated employees in these services are trained in its use and encouraged to use the system as the principal mechanism for searching and accessing medical center documents. The program itself counts each access in order to monitor frequency of use and allow analysis of usage trends. Data gathering continues, and the team expects to assess the process shortly to develop further improvements based on new technology and on what it learns from this experience and from customer feedback.

Author: Rosa Franco graduated from Hunter College, City University of New York with a bachelor's degree in psychology. She began working in VHA in 1987 as the equal employment opportunity manager, a position she held until she became executive assistant for TQI at the New York City VA medical center in 1992.

Access to Policies and Procedures Team

The need to manage paperwork is a recurrent theme in VHA's TQI activities. This team employed a principle we saw over and over in its heavy emphasis on a customer focus. The team also employed a principle that is often associated with high-performing organizations—benchmarking. One measure of their success is the interest that their improvements generated in other VA medical facilities.

In 1993, the quality leadership council of the White City, Oregon, VA domiciliary chartered an improvement team to improve employee access to facility policies and procedures. At that time there were 330 policies and procedures, requiring approximately eighty thousand pages of copying. Complete sets of these documents were found only in selected offices and were generally unavailable to the average employee. Approval time for new policies often took up to ninety days, and copying costs were considered excessive.

The team was led by the executive assistant for TQI; key members were Charles Osborne, Ray Sullivan, and Sandy Preston. Other members included representatives from the medicine, nursing, housekeeping, social work, library, and administrative support services, the information unit, and the director's office. Several team members had served on improvement teams in the past. The team was trained together over a two-day period, using the second day to establish the team's goals and work plan for the project.

The team began benchmarking with other government agencies and private companies, and these contacts provided ideas for a format for rewriting the facility's policies and procedures. It became evident through these benchmarking activities that a revision of the current procedures for initiating and revising policies (shuffling paperwork differently, if you will) would not yield the expected outcomes called for in the team's charter. Further analysis found that policies and procedures were often redundant and described procedures that were either not adhered to or were not uniform throughout the domiciliary. The team returned to the leadership council with a proposal that the entire policy and procedure system be converted to an electronic format integrated with the centralized database for easy access by all employees. Once this idea was approved, the team found a software company that had a potential product and the willingness to modify it to meet the desired objective. Additionally, the team kept close and continuous contact with the internal customers in designing the format, content, and information-retrieval features of the new system.

Over a twelve-month period, the team not only converted the policy and procedure system to a centralized process but also achieved the following results:

- All policies and procedures were made instantly available to all employees. The team provided the necessary training to service representatives using a "train-the-trainer" approach.
- Concurrence time for policy and procedures was reduced from two to three months to ten days.
- A 100 percent reduction in copying was achieved, yielding an annual savings of approximately $26,000.
- Redundancy among documents was reduced dramatically. Total policies and procedures were reduced from 330 to 200.
- Clinical and off-tour administrative personnel now have immediate access to facility decision-making procedures through a system with appropriate search capabilities.
- Policies and procedures now average 56 lines (one page), compared to an average of 205 lines (four pages) prior to the improvement.

This improvement initiative has to date been shared with approximately eighty other VA hospitals, as well as several private facilities. The initiative provided lasting and impressive improvements for the domiciliary. The team was nationally recognized with the vice president's Hammer Award in September 1994.

Author: Jeff Bellah has been the executive assistant for quality management at the White City domiciliary since 1989. He was the author of the application that won the Robert W. Carey Quality Award in 1995.

Administrative Processes with Clinical Implications
Availability of Clean Beds Team

TQI practitioners often hear about the importance of stakeholders and the need to keep them aware of and involved in the improvement process. This team illustrates how early resistance was overcome by focusing on a major stakeholder. Another important lesson in this story is the effective use of the plan, do, check, act cycle in process improvement. Teams are often tempted to jump to the "act" part of the cycle without adequately performing the "do" and "study" functions. This team resisted that temptation, and by doing so it was able to overcome early resistance before hospital-wide implementation.

One of the initial assessment teams at the Olin E. Teague VA medical center in Temple, Texas, reviewed the patient admission process and identified availability of clean beds as an opportunity for improvement. The assessment team found that patient beds, including intensive care beds, were not being cleaned in a timely manner following the discharge or transfer of patients; this problem had a significant impact on the timeliness of new admissions.

As a result of the team's findings, the quality leadership team (QLT) formally chartered a process action team (PAT) to examine the process from the time a patient is discharged from a bed until the time the same bed is ready for a new patient. The team charter was developed by the QLT in May 1993. The QLT selected Ms. Darlene Neiser, R.N., a quality management program assistant, as the team leader and Ms. Karen Robbins, Psy.D., a staff psychologist, as the team facilitator. The team leader then collaborated with a QLT representative in choosing the most appropriate team members. Team membership included representatives from the nursing service, the environmental management service (EMS), and the medical administration service (MAS).

The PAT attended a three-day team training course in June 1993 presented by two consultants from the American Productivity and Quality Center (APQC). During this training, the team quickly recognized that the initial goal of reviewing the process from discharge until a new patient is placed in the bed involved a bed-control process and a bed-cleaning process. The team narrowed the focus of the charter to "improving the process of getting a vacated bed cleaned and notifying MAS that the bed is available." The change in the original charter was approved by the QLT.

The PAT members surveyed the various patient care areas responsible for patient admissions as to their specific bed-cleaning process, resulting in a flowchart of the process for each area. The team then combined them into one large macro flowchart depicting how the process was actually working. The flowchart included routine and stat methods of bed cleaning during administrative and nonadministrative hours. The complexity of the existing process is illustrated by a portion of that flowchart, shown in Figure 12.5.

The team also completed a *process definition sheet* and a *requirements definition sheet* identifying and analyzing the key components of the process (inputs, outputs, customers, suppliers, and customer requirements). Through flowcharting the current process and talking to employees directly involved in it, the team discovered that a defined bed-cleaning procedure did not exist for any area in the medical center. Furthermore, the team discovered that the patient units used informal, unwritten signals (for example, raising or lowering the head or foot of a bed) to indicate that something needed to be done or a task on the bed had been completed. Complicating matters even further, these signals meant different things on different units and during different shifts. The team also discovered that nursing personnel were removing and disposing of the soiled linen and then applying clean linen once the bed unit had been cleaned by EMS staff. (A "bed unit" consists of a bed, nightstand, overbed table, overhead light, chairs, floor, and locker.)

For two months, the team tracked the number of beds cleaned in each unit and identified whether they were cleaned due to patient discharges or patient transfers. They did this by collecting log sheets from the EMS staff which identified the number of bed units cleaned. This was done in order to identify overall work load and also to identify those wards with a high volume of cleaning. The surgical service was found to have the highest volume of beds requiring cleaning. However, the medicine service was the only section with an assigned bed cleaner. During the data collection period, the treatment team identified a problem with the patient transfer process. While this issue was related to the bed-cleaning process, it was outside the scope of the team's mission. The team referred this issue to the nursing service for resolution.

Upon the completion of the data collection, the PAT constructed a cause-and-effect diagram. Specific causes identified by the team included the lack of a policy and procedure for bed cleaning, insufficient bed-cleaning staff assigned to the acute medicine bed section (there was only one full-time bed cleaner), a lack of available pagers, inadequate communication, and the lack of an

Figure 12.5. Bed-Cleaning Process.

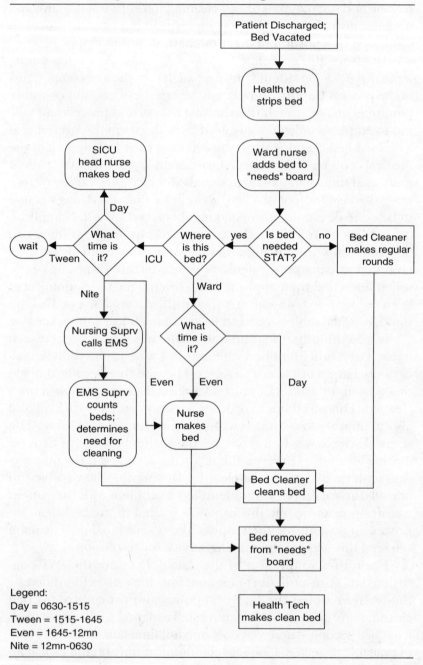

Legend:
Day = 0630-1515
Tween = 1515-1645
Even = 1645-12mn
Nite = 12mn-0630

automated tracking and notification system. The PAT surveyed approximately twenty other VA medical centers, gathering information about the use of computer programs for communication, the assignment of bed cleaner positions, service responsibility, issues concerning bed linens, and bed-cleaning policies and procedures. Additionally, the team reviewed various DHCP applications that offered potential solutions to the communication process. However, except for regular E-mail, the programs all proved to be too cumbersome and created additional work.

The PAT worked closely with the chief of EMS and the chief of the nursing service to develop a policy and procedure for twenty-four-hour-coverage bed-cleaning services for the medicine and surgery services, including the intensive care unit. The new procedure assigned responsibility to nursing personnel to remove all supplies, medical equipment, and patient effects from the room upon discharge of the patient. The ward clerk would notify EMS of the vacant bed and whether or not it was a priority (a "priority" bed is a vacant bed in one of the intensive care wards or a bed on any ward needed for a waiting patient). The bed-cleaning staff would then clean the beds in the order notified, except for priority beds. Bed cleaner responsibilities now include removing and disposing of soiled linen, cleaning the bed unit, and applying clean linen. In December 1993, a pilot study of the new procedure was conducted with bed cleaners assigned to medicine and surgery bed sections. Each bed cleaner was issued a pager. PAT members provided one-on-one, intensive in-service training with unit staff on all three tours, clarifying the process and identifying present and potential problems. The PAT was surprised to find initial implementation of the process "shaky" due to resistance to change and turf issues. Nursing and EMS staff needed clarification, support, and encouragement to make the changes work. Additional explanation and education was provided for staff on all three tours, with discussion concerning benefits of the change for staff and resulting positive impact on patient care.

At the completion of the pilot, a final version of the policy and procedure was created. A monitoring tool to measure the effectiveness of the new process was also developed. Each month, thirty beds are randomly selected for inspection by the EMS supervisor. The supervisor checks to be sure that the supplies and patient effects are removed by nursing staff and that the bed and bed unit are completely cleaned and ready for occupancy. The results are then reported on a quarterly basis at EMS staff meetings. In March 1994, the PAT's recommendations were approved by the QLT. The medical center now has a standard method of bed cleaning for patient care units with designated bed cleaners. An additional improvement included a change to fitted sheets in order to standardize linen preparation across units.

Through this experience the PAT identified a problem with adequate discharge planning. The lack of a standardized discharge time was a major contributor to discharges occurring late in the day. In response to these findings, the QLT chartered a discharge planning process improvement team.

The monitoring tool shows that the process is working well and staff complaints have significantly decreased. While the process is not completely problem-free, issues are now continuously dealt with when they occur. Elvis Thomas, the housekeeping supervisor for EMS, summed the situation up in his comment, "Before we started TQI, it would take approximately thirty to forty-five minutes per individual to get a bed cleaned from the time EMS was notified of a vacant bed. But since the changes with TQI, now the average time from notification until the bed is ready to be occupied is twenty minutes, while priority beds average ten minutes. This leaves nurses to do other things rather than making beds."

Author: Ron Weaver received his undergraduate degree from Rhodes College in 1980, and he earned a master's degree in both health care administration and business administration at the University of Mississippi in 1983. He has worked in the VA health care system for twelve years. Most recently, he was the administrative assistant to the chief of staff at the Olin E. Teague veterans center before he became executive assistant for TQI.

"Drugs 'R' Us" Team

Inherent in TQI is the establishment of teams that bring together groups of staff who often do not normally work together. A not-unexpected outcome is turmoil. Overcoming turmoil, therefore, is an important feature of the team process. Sometimes teams must stop what they are doing and address tur-

moil directly. This team did just that, and a successful outcome was the re-sult. This team also illustrates how the simple tools of TQI, such as flow-charting, can be significant eye-openers.

The Dayton, Ohio, VA medical center is very proud of its "Drugs 'R' Us" process action team, which received the vice president's 1994 Hammer Award for excellence in reinventing government. This team was chartered in December 1992 by the quality council after sixty-three complaints of drug outages were received in one month from patients and clinicians. Team members from the acquisition and materiel management service (A&MMS) and the pharmacy service were asked to evaluate and improve the drug acquisition process, beginning with the clinician's order and ending when the drug was made available to the patient.

During the two and a half days of training provided for this team, emphasis was placed on team building, individual and team empowerment, TQI principles, TQI tools, and process improvement as it relates to the ordering and procurement process. Although the common stages of team growth—"forming, storming, norming, and performing," as described by Peter Scholtes in *The Team Handbook* (1988, pp. 1–4)—were discussed, the team members did not expect it to be a problem they would encounter.

This team experienced both challenges and personal growth while dealing with the issue of drug outages. The nine-member team contained a mixture of volunteers and individuals selected by their service chief. The team leader was John Roberts, a general supply specialist from A&MMS, and the team facilitator was Suzanne Schrand, a statistics clerk from the medical administration service (MAS). Service chiefs from A&MMS and the pharmacy service were appointed as joint process owners and attended the team training.

As a result of the team's training, several process-related issues became apparent. Each service felt that "the other guys" needed a lot of improvement. Multiple purchase orders were created in emergencies, costing more in both dollars and staff time. The two services did not understand each other's roles, leading to many episodes of blaming and finger-pointing. All the time the team was chartered, the advent of VHA's "Prime Vendor" pharmacy program (a centralized clearinghouse and distribution plan for pharmaceutical products) was rumored to be "just around the corner." Team members were concerned that their work and effort might be for nothing if the process they redesigned was replaced by this program. It soon became apparent, however, that major improvements in the current process were mandatory even to adapt to the Prime Vendor program.

The flowcharting process was an eye-opener for all involved. The drug delivery process was extremely complicated, convoluted, and lengthy. Multiple steps were identified as valueless and repetitive, especially inspection steps (1–4 below) that were layered one upon the other and sprinkled liberally throughout.

Figure 12.6. Excerpt from the "Drugs 'R' Us" Team Flowchart.

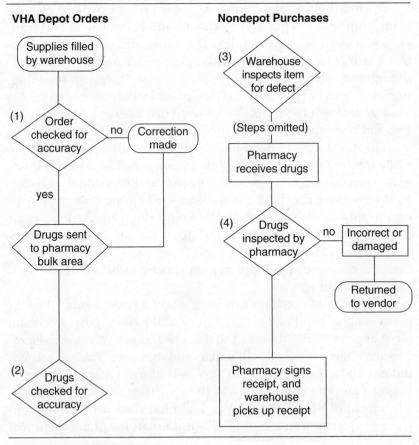

Some parts of the process could not be flowcharted initially due to the amount of variation or confusion about "the way it was done." The commitment of individual team members was evident from the beginning as they developed measurement strategies, cross-trained one another, discussed problem areas, and benchmarked with other organizations. The group soon fell into a lively storming stage. Issues of turf, blame, fear of changing roles, and fear of job loss—whether justified or not—led to a group that functioned in a very antagonistic manner. Interestingly, the team made considerable progress even during this storming stage.

To assist the team in resolving the conflict and to improve the group process, the team facilitator held a training session to discuss the issue. The real breakthrough came when one team member began a meeting by stating that she had not been following the team rules of trust; she vowed to do so from then on, and she asked the others to join her. This change in attitude was adopted by other members and they became a real *team* rather than just a group. Within four months the team made recommendations that resulted in the following improvements:

- Reduction in the time required to deliver drugs from the A&MMS warehouse to the pharmacy from 3.5 hours to 14 minutes
- Elimination and consolidation of duplicate inventories in the pharmacy, resulting in better inventory control
- Cross-training between pharmacy and A&MMS staff in both inventory control and ordering processes
- Reduction in posted stock inventory, which resulted in a savings of $139,849
- Reduction in the number of drug outages by 91 percent
- Substantially improved communication between the services

As stated earlier, the Dayton facility is very proud of these two services and of the team members, who completed a difficult task while showing that real teamwork can overcome many barriers.

Author: Charlene Marbury, R.N., B.S., M.H.A, is the TQI coordinator at Dayton. Marbury came to VHA in 1983 as an infection control coordinator, transferred to quality management, and in 1992 was selected as TQI coordinator.

Medical Records Availability Team

TQI practitioners are enjoined to break processes down into manageable parts in search of root causes. Teams often encounter easily solved problems and are sometimes sidetracked by the "obvious fix." At VHA, we often call this "peeling the onion." The lesson is a simple one, but nonetheless one that is often ignored: do not get caught up fixing a lot of little things when there may be a root cause whose solution will have a greater impact.

Medical records availability was identified through an employee survey at the Reno, Nevada, VA medical center as one of the key processes that needed improvement in order to meet the center's "critical success factors." Thus, a process action team was launched in July 1992. The goal of this team was to increase medical records availability to clinics. Through flowcharting the process, several problem areas were identified, such as medical records being utilized for reasons other than direct patient care (for example, for quality assurance reviews and research), daily clinic add-ons, the bottleneck created when an expeditor is needed to find charts that are not available, lack of timeliness in returning charts to the file room, and the current practice by some programs of keeping the chart throughout a treatment process that might take weeks or months. These processes were then evaluated through the use of a cause-and-effect diagram, shown in Figure 12.7.

This process narrowed the concerns about records not being located in the file room to charts not being recharged, inadequate tracking, and records not being returned to the file room. Several methods were used to collect data around these concerns. These included surveys, interviews, chart reviews, logging time frames in the process, and focus groups.

The findings of the data collection process revealed a very complex process with many potential areas for improvement. A thorough review and prioritization of these issues found that ultimately the root cause was the current record storage and retrieval process itself, which was unable to physically meet the demands placed on it by medical center staff. That is to say, a record often needs to be in more than one place at the same time, because different staff have legitimate needs for it at the same time. We concluded that a computerized medical records process was needed in order to provide information in a timely and accurate manner. Because the

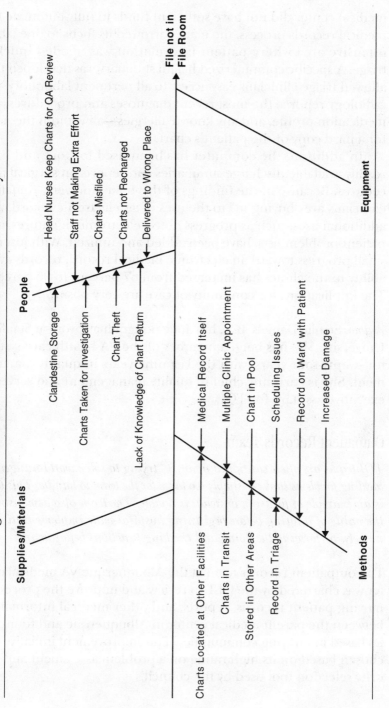

Figure 12.7. Reasons for Medical Records Unavailability.

Supplies/Materials

People

File not in File Room

Head Nurses Keep Charts for QA Review

Clandestine Storage

Staff not Making Extra Effort

Charts Taken for Investigation

Charts Misfiled

Chart Theft

Charts not Recharged

Lack of Knowledge of Chart Return

Delivered to Wrong Place

Equipment

Medical Record Itself

Multiple Clinic Appointment

Chart in Pool

Scheduling Issues

Record on Ward with Patient

Increased Damage

Charts Located at Other Facilities

Charts in Transit

Stored in Other Areas

Record in Triage

Methods

medical center did not have sufficient funds to fully automate the medical records process, the team narrowed its focus to one labor-intensive area where patient information was needed quickly: triage. A specific computerized health summary was developed that allowed triage clinicians easy access to all pertinent laboratory and radiology reports, the most recent diagnoses and procedures, the medication profile, and any known allergies—all without the need for a hard copy of the patient's chart.

In addition, the computer has been used to store and have readily available discharge summaries and reports on surgical procedures. Because of the findings of this team, formerly reluctant clinicians are "buying in" to the uses of an electronic record; and additional uses, such as progress notes, electronic signatures, and patient problem lists, have been added and utilized. With just this small progress toward an electronic medical record, records availability to the clinics has increased from 67 percent to 96 percent. The implications for continuity of care are very positive.

Author: Stanlie Daniels, B.S., has done postgraduate work at Stanford University. She has been a member of the VA health care system for twenty-four years, with the last nine years in quality management. She is currently chief of quality management and serves as executive assistant for TQI.

Outpatient Records Team

TQI teams are often cautioned against "trying to solve world hunger" by tackling problems that are simply too large for the team to handle. This team is an example of focusing on what is doable. The team also demonstrates the value of piloting before beginning hospital-wide implementation— namely, performing the doing and checking functions before acting.

The outpatient records team at the Albuquerque VA medical center was chartered by the QLT to review and improve the process of moving patient records, reports, and other medical information between the parent medical center in Albuquerque and four clinics based in outlying communities. This improvement initiative was chosen based on its high rating on a problem assessment and priority selection tool used by the council.

The team included representatives from nursing, clinical representation from the managed care section, laboratory, representation from the medical staff, social work staff, and administrative support service. The team leader was a nurse representative from the managed care section, and the facilitator was from the media production service. As the team progressed toward implementing a solution, additional representatives were included.

The team began their process improvement journey by collecting data regarding return of records following appointments or hospitalization at the Albuquerque medical center. Analyzing the inpatient and outpatient record transfer process using a flowchart was the next step. This enabled the team to narrow its improvement efforts to the outpatient record transfer process. The team used a cause-and-effect diagram, which clearly demonstrated a lack of a consistent method for moving records and information.

Three improvements were recommended by the team. First, the name of the appropriate community clinic was placed on patients' cards to help identify where to return reports. Second, a new process was put in place to expedite the movement of patient records between outlying clinics and the Albuquerque medical center. Third, a health benefits adviser was added to the process to coordinate and track the process. The new process was successfully piloted in one community clinic and is now used in all four community clinics. Color-coded medical records are now used as an additional method of identifying the outlying clinics, and space in the file room is specifically allocated for these clinic charts.

Data gathered for six months in 1994 showed an 84 percent availability rate for medical records, which was a significant improvement over previous rates. Other results were easier identification of clinic records and an improved method for transferring records.

The team worked for almost a year on this initiative. The administrative support staff have taken over ownership of the process and continue to improve the work of the team.

Author: Michael Sergent is the executive assistant for TQI at the Albuquerque VA medical center. He has worked for the Department of Veterans Affairs for twenty-four years. Prior to 1991, Sergent worked in mental health. He holds a bachelor's degree in psychology from California State University, San Jose, and a master's degree in marriage, family, and child counseling from Santa Clara University.

Clinical Issues Involving Administrative Processes

Admissions Process Team

This team's activities illustrate several TQI truisms. First, team champions are important to a team's success, and they can come from anywhere in the organization. Here the champion was an admissions clerk whose work would be directly affected by the outcome. Also, early team successes generate enthusiasm, and TQI teams should strive for early success to maintain momentum. Finally, unanticipated benefits often arise when teams study the outcomes of process changes.

The VA medical center in Dallas, Texas, formally embarked on its implementation of TQI in the fall of 1992. Before that date the center had established several informal quality improvement teams, and in September 1992 it began using a strategic process improvement model to identify and address opportunities for improvement.

One of the ten major improvement processes targeted by the QLT was the admissions process. Based on past practice and general knowledge, the QLT decided that improving this process would have a major impact on improving customer satisfaction, reducing duplication of effort, and streamlining a cross-functional activity.

A process improvement team was established to assess the current admissions process. The administrative assistant for the surgical service, the nurse manager of the day surgery unit, and the assistant chief of the medical service were selected to conduct the assessment. Focus group interviews were held with patients and facility staff to determine what they liked and did not like about the current admissions process. The assessment report noted, "We find the process to be unacceptable. Customer complaints are frequent. There is no apparent measurement of the process, and in its current state the overall process is costly. There is no standard policy related to utilization of bed assignments and admissions personnel." The assessment also revealed that patients were spending considerable time and energy completing the admissions process. "[The patient] moves through the system, going from first floor, to second floor, to the basement, back to the first floor, and then to the assigned bed . . . and [the patient] is the one with the medical problem." The average scheduled admission took two and a half hours to complete.

Based on the findings of the assessment team, the scheduled admissions process was one of the first quality improvement initiatives to be chartered by the leadership council. The team leader was Burlean Huff. Other team members included a representative from the administrative support service, a supervisor for ward clerks, an admissions clerk (the true champion of the improvement initiative), a nurse manager from the day surgery unit, and a clerk from radiology. Representation from involved service units proved to be a key factor in the team's success. Because of the volatility of the process and the possibility of territorial issues, Jeff Burk, the strong, knowledgeable assistant chief of the psychology service, was selected to serve as facilitator. This task tested the facilitator's skills as counselor, mediator, and peacemaker.

The team leader and facilitator attended a one-day training session, which was followed by a two-day team training session. The spirit of the team was captured in their rules of operation—they named themselves "the A Team" and vowed not to progress through any "storming" stages.

The team was charged to improve the scheduled admissions process by reducing the number of tasks and the distance patients must go from the point of checking in at the admissions desk until they arrive at their assigned bed. The team was determined to approach the process from the patient's point of view. This was accomplished by having team members follow patients. The patients most frequently complained that the process was too long and that they were asked the same questions repeatedly. The team solicited input from each professional group involved in the process. Figure 12.8 shows part of the team's flowchart of the admissions process.

The team's enthusiasm increased as they identified early improvements from their recommendations and as they achieved "buy-in" from key groups. The team reported to the leadership

Figure 12.8. Baseline Patient Admitting Steps.

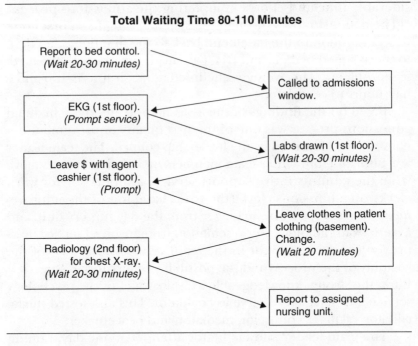

Total Waiting Time 80-110 Minutes

Report to bed control.
(Wait 20-30 minutes)

Called to admissions window.

EKG (1st floor).
(Prompt service)

Labs drawn (1st floor).
(Wait 20-30 minutes)

Leave $ with agent cashier (1st floor).
(Prompt)

Leave clothes in patient clothing (basement). Change.
(Wait 20 minutes)

Radiology (2nd floor) for chest X-ray.
(Wait 20-30 minutes)

Report to assigned nursing unit.

council in four months, requesting permission to pilot their recommendations. A one-month pilot study was conducted, with overwhelming success.

Improvements made in the scheduled admissions process include:

- Changes in the clinic where patients are scheduled for admission. Patients are given an admission instruction sheet informing them of their admission date and time, the name of their provider, and what to bring with them to the hospital.
- A uniform admission order form for both medical and surgical patients.
- Combining the functions of utilization control and admissions, thereby eliminating a step in the process.
- Providing for the completion of necessary radiology work-ups on the first floor. This recommendation has resulted in a cost

savings, as the center no longer performs routine chest X-rays on preoperative and medical admissions.

- Delaying the drawing of laboratory specimens until the patient has been admitted to the unit. This eliminated another step in the admissions process. Since admissions are done with greater expediency, the patients are on the unit in time for the afternoon laboratory team to draw the specimens.
- Encouraging patients to bring their own pajamas, slippers, and robes. This eliminates the visit to the clothing room. Pajamas are now stocked on all nursing units. If a patient does have luggage, staff from the facility deliver it to the clothing room until the patient is discharged.

Several unanticipated improvements have been realized as a result of the new process. The dietary service no longer has to deliver late meals, as patients are on the unit in ample time to get meals at the regular time. The center no longer orders as many pajamas, since patients are wearing their own. The admissions area waiting room is less congested, as patients are being processed much quicker.

It has been two years since the center implemented the new process, and the scheduled admissions team continues to realize its goals. In some cases as many as five process steps have been eliminated. Duplication and rework have been reduced. The most obvious benefit has been the reduction in the average time of admission from two and a half hours to less than thirty minutes. Internal and external customer satisfaction has improved. Patients continue to be amazed and grateful for the changes.

Author: Gail Bentley, Ph.D, R.N., is currently the associate chief of staff for education at the Dallas VA medical center. She was appointed as the executive assistant for TQI in July 1992 and continues to serve in that role.

Hospital-Based Home Care Team

This team is an example of a service-level initiative, common in VA hospitals. Once TQI has been implemented hospital-wide, usually by teams that cross service and functional lines, individual services or units often embark on their own TQI activities. This team made improvements within its own

*sphere of activity, piloted those improvements, and recommended applica-
tion of the improvements in other services.*

In the spring of 1993, the Minneapolis VA medical center formally
launched its quality improvement journey by conducting an organizational leadership conference in which the director challenged
staff to identify quality improvement initiatives. The staff of the
hospital-based home care (HBHC) program accepted this challenge and requested the assistance of a RMEC master trainer to assist us in exploring opportunities to improve our program.

The entire HBHC staff participated in a one-day workshop to
learn the principles and techniques of process improvement. The
outcome of the day's activities was an assessment that indicated that
a proper admissions assessment, patient education, coordination
of care, and management of medical conditions were key processes. From this list, patient assessment was selected as a priority
improvement, as problems had been identified with this process,
and it seemed amenable to change. The process improvement
team consisted of a physician, Don Masler, who was the team
leader; a RMEC master trainer, who served as facilitator; a nurse;
a social worker; a dietitian; and a rehabilitation technician. The
team went through a two-day training course, which included instruction on key process improvement tools such as flowcharts and
cause-and-effect diagrams.

As a result of this improvement initiative, the team developed
a model for integrating and computerizing independent databases
into a single database. The new system was pilot-tested for six
months, with the following results:

- A reduction in the duplication of assessment information in
  medical center documents. Minimizing duplication resulted in
  an annual savings of over 120 hours of staff time in data entry
  alone. Projecting these savings across all members of the program staff would result in a savings of approximately 627
  hours annually.
- Development of a streamlined approach to service delivery.
  This resulted in increased productivity and improved program
  staff morale.

- The time spent on this initiative generated a greater respect for the contributions of the various disciplines and a new sense of "team."

The team prepared a final report outlining the pilot improvement results, including a recommendation that the new assessment data collection methodology be extended to other clinical systems outside the HBHC. The team also requested laptop computers with modems, which would allow the HBHC staff access to a full range of medical center data from patients' homes.

Author: Tom Sullivan, M.S.W., A.C.S.W., Lic. S.W., served as the chair of the hospital-based home care database team. Tom also has served as facilitator for other process improvement groups within the medical center. He has been with the Department of Veterans Affairs since 1985.

Outpatient Timeliness Team

This story illustrates how a team can successfully tackle a large issue and, over time, make improvements. The key to the team's success can be seen in the way it methodically and patiently addressed each part of the bigger issue. Simple solutions often resolved chronic problems.

The Pathfinders, so named because it was the first process improvement team established at the Big Spring, Texas, VA medical center, was chartered in April 1992 by the chief of staff. Top management and staff had long been aware of the excessive time required for a veteran to complete an outpatient visit, but this was the first formal attempt to solicit input from the real subject matter experts—the employees on the front line. A ten-member, multidisciplinary team was selected from a wide range of hospital services—administrative support, pharmacy, nursing, medicine, radiology, and laboratory. The team also included a patient representative and two representatives from the veteran patient population.

The Pathfinder's goals were to decrease waiting time for walk-in patients, ensure that scheduled patients were seen on time, and improve employee morale and patient satisfaction. To these ends, the team was charged with reviewing the entire general medicine outpatient clinic admissions process and all processes that had an impact on timeliness.

The team began by defining their purpose, exploring what they knew about customers and suppliers, and determining action plans based on analyses of process data. Data collected included a list of the most frequent reasons for appointment delays, the number and types of patients on each day of the week, which times of the day were most active, the number of prescriptions filled for each type of patient, the average waiting time for a prescription to be filled, daily statistics on the length of patient visits (walk-in and by appointment), usage patterns for patient care area space and equipment, an analysis of available patient waiting areas, and an in-depth review of locally established policies and procedures to determine if any were causing bottlenecks in the process. The relatively mundane review of local policies uncovered interesting problems. For example, Big Spring had a policy that allowed the pharmacy to accept only original signatures on prescription forms. The prescription forms used at Big Spring consisted of an original and two carbon copies. Patients often took the carbon copy to the pharmacy and were turned away to get an original signature. The simple solution was to retain the original in the medical record and have the pharmacy accept any legible carbon copy. Also, legibility of handwriting was an issue on prescriptions. The team recommended training for physicians on this issue, which included information on the problems encountered by staff.

As a result of their data analysis, the team recommended improvement initiatives to decrease waiting times for prescriptions, reduce paperwork, implement primary care models, and realign administrative duties in the outpatient care area. The implementation of primary care involved a redesign of the physical layout. The area had previously been an admissions ward; it was broken into many small rooms where clinicians provided care to patients, who went from room to room. The team redesigned the area so that patients would be directed to a single room, where the providers would come to them. Other design changes included placing the travel clerk, cashier, and pharmacy (all stops made at the end of the process) adjacent to one another.

These initiatives have resulted in a decrease in total processing time from four hours and forty-two minutes in June 1992 to two hours and fifty-seven minutes in June 1993. In addition, the increased efficiencies derived from these improvements decreased overtime during 1993, with a financial savings of $56,447.

Author: JoAnne Staulkup is a computer specialist whose previous duties included chief of the ambulatory care and processing section. She has served with the Department of Veterans Affairs for twenty-nine years.

Outpatient Clinic Team

There is a cliche that goes, "If it ain't broke, don't fix it." This cliche does not necessarily apply to TQI. Key members of this team did not agree that the process they examined needed fixing. In fact, there was initial reluctance to participate because of that perception. After studying their process, however, the team members came to a realization that even if the process was not broken, it could still be improved, and the time spent making the improvements was worth the effort. In fact, it was that realization by team members that galvanized their improvement efforts.

As health system specialist for ambulatory care at the VA medical center in Lexington, Kentucky, I was the first point of contact for the executive assistant for TQI organizing a new process improvement team. My initial reaction to this inquiry was similar to the reaction of parents when told their child has done something wrong. While I recognized the fact that our ambulatory care program was not perfect, I certainly didn't like someone else pointing out our flaws. My negative reaction was compounded by the fact that I had had a less-than-positive experience on two other improvement teams. I was convinced, based on these past experiences, that TQI was too slow and did not necessarily change anything. Fortunately, I suppressed this initial reaction and cheerfully responded with, "Sure, that sounds like a great idea. We always want to improve things in our area. I'd love to be on the team." The challenge of analyzing a system and finding ways to improve it did indeed interest me.

It was with these somewhat mixed emotions that I began my

journey on TQI Process Improvement Team 16. The journey began in July 1993 and continues to this day as part of the ambulatory care service's ongoing customer service efforts. The original improvement team was initiated by the quality leadership council, based on a recommendation from another team that had assessed patient satisfaction. With input from the associate chief of staff for ambulatory care, the executive assistant for TQI and I selected the team membership, which included the outpatient clinic nurse manager, an administrative clerk, an outpatient social worker, an internal medicine physician, and a facilitator, Phyllis Barrett, R.N. Like me, each of these individuals brought with them varying biases as well as assets.

The outpatient clinic nurse manager, Jerry Karr, R.N., served as team leader. Since he had been a staff nurse for a number of years, he knew the ins and outs of the system. However, he was also convinced that we didn't have any problems, citing the fact that the area where the delays occurred was the admissions and evaluation area, not the outpatient clinic area. Our physician representative was an experienced health systems researcher. He made sure our team acted on statistically significant data. The social work representative and the facilitator were less familiar with the processing of patients in the outpatient clinic, but they were able to give slightly different perspectives that balanced the views of those more involved with the process. We were also fortunate to have the input of a computer programmer, who worked closely with our team to create a mechanism for obtaining data from the system.

Early team meetings involved defining and redefining the team's goals. The team had been given a fairly broad charter, to improve timeliness. One of the boundaries to that charter called for the process to end at the time medications were dispensed from the pharmacy, and the team spent a great deal of time questioning that boundary. Also, the charge called for the team to look at patient profiles, but the team decided not to do so because the information was not useful. Next came the somewhat arduous process of constructing flowcharts. While these initial phases took considerable time, they allowed rapport to develop among the group, and they set the stage for our future team interactions.

After these phases were accomplished, we began to ask ourselves what information or data we needed to assess the delays. We decided that there were really two parallel issues regarding delays: (1) patient perceptions of the outpatient experience and (2) actual processing times. We needed data on both issues. We developed a patient satisfaction survey and a time study, and we worked with computer staff to develop a computer program to monitor processing times by clinic staff. Using quality improvement tools, we analyzed the data and formulated recommendations. Our recommendations ranged from minor changes that we were able to implement as we went along to continuous monitoring activities. In essence, we learned that overall outpatient clinic processing times were not too bad, but there was room to improve both patient perceptions and actual processing time. Figure 12.9 shows a control chart (adapted from an actual chart showing over thirty clinics) listing average times for specific outpatient clinics.

This chart shows that waiting times were generally within control limits. The realization by team members that although waiting times were in control, improvements could still be made was a key to the success of the team, and we did accomplish several things:

- Changes in patient appointment letters and improved communication with patients
- Creation of provider-specific clinics to enhance scheduling practices
- Provision of patient education materials to make waiting times more productive
- Increased staff sensitivity to the issue of patient waiting times
- Creation of a computer program to help monitor patient waiting times and to position ourselves for compliance with customer service standards
- Changed practices in one outlying clinic to reduce needless waits for laboratory tests

The process improvement team presented its final report as part of our JCAHO survey in June 1995. The surveyors were extremely impressed with the teamwork and enthusiasm involved in the effort.

Author: Charlene Gathy holds a master's degree in public administration. She has been with the Department of Veterans Affairs

Figure 12.9. Control Chart for Outpatient Waiting Times.

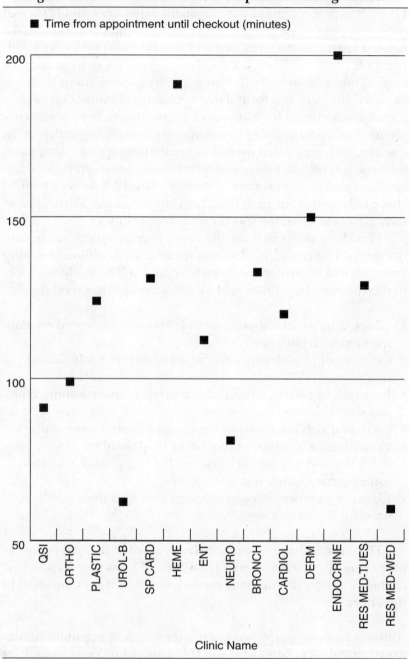

since 1986 and has been a health system specialist for ambulatory care for four years.

Processes with a Direct Clinical Impact
Transporting Patients Team

This story illustrates a number of features that appeared in prior team stories and one that did not: namely, a call for volunteers to staff the team. The team's refocusing of its charter is by now a familiar theme, and we are reminded again of the critical role of "buy-in" by stakeholders.

In July 1993, the QLT at the Loma Linda VA medical center chartered a new cross-functional team to examine the issue of transporting patients within the medical center. The impetus for this charter came from two sources. First, there had been recent reports of incidents involving the transport of critically ill patients for tests. Second, one of the physician members of the QLT was responsible for the intensive care unit, and some of the incidents involved patients under his care. That physician became the team's sponsor.

Critically ill patients often need highly specialized therapeutic and diagnostic procedures that are not available on their wards. Thus, they often need to be transported to, and returned from, various areas of the hospital where such procedures are available. Because of the severity of their medical condition, they must be transported along with various lifesaving appurtenances, such as intravenous bags, drainage tubes, and lifesaving equipment and medications, and they must be transported by staff trained in the use of that equipment and those medications and knowledgeable about various lifesaving techniques. Mary Anne Collins, a nurse educator and team facilitator, points out that "taking emergency drugs with critically ill patients is a community standard of care. Further, the Joint Commission on Accreditation of Healthcare Organizations requires that patients receive the same quality of care while being transported as they would receive on their critical care ward." The team's first step was to advertise the charter hospitalwide and ask all interested employees to apply for team membership. The final selection of the team members was made by the QLT using selection criteria and a matrix.

Team members included Karen Pierce, a nurse manager, who was the team leader; Mary Anne Collins, a nurse educator, who was team facilitator; a hospital volunteer; a medical administration service lead clerk; a pharmacist; and a cook.

When first written, the team's charter read, "To ensure timely coordinated inpatient transportation by qualified staff." After an initial assessment, the team recommended reducing the scope of the charter and submitted the following to the QLT for approval: "To ensure safe, timely, and coordinated transportation of critically ill inpatients by qualified staff for testing." During August 1993, the team was given TQI team training.

In order to develop information on where patients were being taken and who was accompanying them, the team developed a survey form to be used by persons transporting patients to and from testing areas. Although the team had worked with the medical intensive care unit's (MICU) head nurse in developing the survey form, her staff did not initially "buy in" to the process. The head nurse was asked to become a member of the team, and the head nurse suggested that a TQI master trainer provide the MICU staff with TQI awareness training. With these two actions, data gathering became more successful. Figure 12.10 shows the results of surveys conducted by the team to determine the locations to which patients were being transported. These data show that the bulk of the patients were being transported for angiograms and CT scans.

Team members also surveyed transport practices in the community and in other VA hospitals. The results helped shape their recommendations. They found that their present equipment was bulky and large. There was no standard policy for transporting critically ill patients. There was no requirement that the nursing staff have advanced cardiac life support (ACLS) certification. The team also recommended an emergency drug kit similar to one seen at another medical center.

The final report of the team to the QLT included photographs that showed examples of the initial problems nursing staff had in moving a patient. The photographs clearly displayed difficulties in placing the existing bulky equipment around the patient while entering an elevator. During the presentation to the QLT, the physician sponsor stated, "We have had this as a chronic problem ever since I became a member of the staff. It is great to see it finally adequately addressed."

Figure 12.10. Where Patients Are Transported.

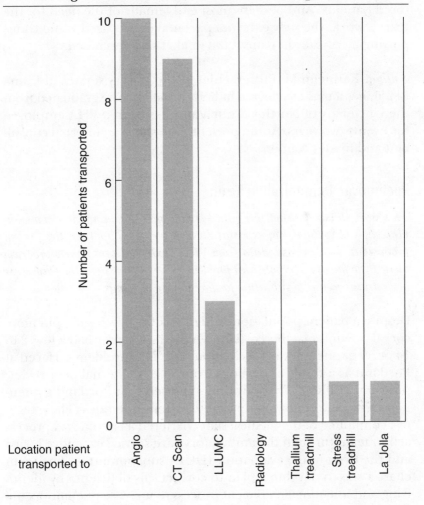

The team's task was completed in July 1994. In June 1995, they checked their results. The equipment for transport was of the same quality as that used in critical care areas. New equipment for use in transporting patients included monitors for blood pressure, pulse, respiration, and oxygen saturation. The new equipment included capabilities for Swan Ganz catheterization, arterial lines, and external pacemaker monitoring. The drug kit was taken on 25 percent of the transports. Eighty-one percent of the staff were

ACLS trained. There was a reduction in the number of unmonitored patients. And perhaps most emblematic of the need for the team's work, the new external pacemaker was used while transporting a critically ill patient the week it was purchased.

Author: Kathleen M. Puffer, chief of the library service at Loma Linda, has a master's degree in library science. She graduated from the University of North Carolina and has been a VHA employee for twenty-two years. At the present time she is an internal consultant and master trainer.

Pneumovax Immunization Team

This story illustrates something that is only now becoming more commonplace in VHA: the use of external data to identify opportunities for improvement. In this case, data from VHA's external peer review program alerted the facility to a potential problem. Also interesting is the team's use of electronic media to substitute for face-to-face meetings.

Despite a patient population at high risk for developing pneumococcal pneumonia, the Portland VA medical center had a low, 2 to 14 percent pneumovax vaccination rate. This problem surfaced at Portland as a result of findings from VHA's external peer review program (EPRP). These findings showed that Portland's pneumovax rates were low compared to systemwide rates. The executive committee of the medical staff chartered a pneumovax process action team through the ambulatory care service executive board and the drug usage evaluation (DUE) subcommittee. The team charter was to develop a plan to correct this deficiency by identifying and initiating an efficient process to increase pneumovax immunization rates and to improve the clinical database regarding pneumovax status.

The team was led by David Nardone, M.D, the assistant chief of staff for ambulatory care, and it was facilitated by the quality management specialist. The team included a representative from the DUE subcommittee, whose interventional study had increased the pneumovax immunization rates to 14 percent—still unacceptably low. Other members included the nursing unit supervisor for the ambulatory care clinics, the automated data processing (ADP) applications coordinator, the pharmacy service ADP coordinator, the inpatient nursing clinical manager, a pharmacy resident, the supervisor for billing and data management, and the administrative support staff supervisor for the clinics.

Meetings began in October 1994 and were held approximately every other week until January 1995. Further discussions were conducted via E-mail until a follow-up meeting in June 1995. The team continues to communicate via E-mail.

The team found that there was no consistent process in place for the administration and documentation of pneumovax immunizations or for assessing patients' pneumovax status. A pilot process was implemented in an ambulatory care general medicine clinic setting with the intent to expand the process throughout all levels of care.

Just-in-time training using the FADE process ("focus, analyze, develop, execute") was provided for the team. The focus phase involved selecting the team, facilitator, recorder, and time keeper. An agenda, team charter, and rules of trust were developed. Finally, guidelines for pneumovax immunization were developed based on a literature review and benchmarking. The analysis phase included initial brainstorming, flowcharting the existing process, brainstorming ideas for desired outcomes, and flowcharting the desired process. The develop phase created an implementation plan that included a pilot project in a general medicine clinic that called for monitoring outcomes. The execute phase called for educating staff on implementation and on monitoring outcomes.

Measurements used in the process included continuous review of DHCP counts to determine the number of patients who received pneumovax at the time of their clinic visit or on a previous visit, as documented on the electronic progress note data entered into DHCP. The team also randomly selected a general medicine clinic single provider, and a specific month to monitor the percentage of immunizations provided. The numerator was the number of high-risk patients seen by a provider who received pneumovax, and the denominator was the number of high-risk patients seen by a provider. The effectiveness of the team's intervention is demonstrated in Table 12.1.

The impact of the improvement process was to improve the clinical outcomes of the targeted population of patients who

**Table 12.1. Comparative Monthly Results,
Pre- and Postintervention.**

1994	1995
02/94 13	02/95 111
03/94 12	03/95 168
04/94 37	04/95 130
05/94 35	05/95 115
06/94 35	06/95 42

needed pneumovax by increasing the number of patients who receive the vaccine. During clinic visits in February 1994, thirteen patients received pneumovax. During clinic visits in May 1995, 115 patients received pneumovax.

Authors: Fran Hardiman is a quality management specialist. She received her B.S.N. degree from the University of Portland. She has worked for VHA for six years and has spent the last four years in her current position. Beth Schaefer is the chief of the quality management and improvement service. She received her M.P.A. degree from the University of Colorado. She has worked for VHA for thirteen years and has spent the last six years in her current position.

Clinical Pathway—Total Hip Replacement Team

This story describes the events leading to one of the early clinical pathways in VHA. It is one of the early examples of a purely clinical application of TQI. The emphasis on measurable outcomes is also noteworthy. TQI efforts such as this resulted in the Albany VA medical center receiving the Robert W. Carey Quality Award in 1993.

Design a clinical pathway for patients receiving primary total hip replacements (THR)—this was the charge given to us by the TQI steering committee at the Samuel S. Stratton VA medical center in Albany, New York, in the spring of 1992. At the same time, we accepted an invitation by the Iroquois Healthcare Consortium to participate in a two-year demonstration project, which included six area hospitals, to develop THR pathways.

We organized a core team, led jointly by Emma Aliwalas, chief of physical medicine and rehabilitation, and Franklin Glockner, chief of the orthopedic section. Our goal was to improve the quality of care, patients' perception of their experience, and hospital efficiency through the collaborative efforts of representatives from many disciplines, including orthopedics, rehabilitative medicine, social work, medical administration, pharmacy, and nursing. In addition, many others were invited to offer their expertise as resource persons throughout the process. The TQI clinical specialist was the team facilitator.

Training sessions in TQI methodology were provided to the team members and the work began. The process of total hip replacement surgery as it had traditionally been provided was studied by gathering data through retrospective chart reviews, preparing an "as is" pathway, and conducting prepathway patient and staff satisfaction surveys. By analyzing the findings, we were able to identify areas that could be improved.

A "should be" pathway was drafted, consisting of an outline of a desired time line for events and sequences of care. The goal of the pathway was to provide a guideline for managed care throughout preadmission, the acute hospital stay, and postdischarge care in order to reach desired outcomes in an efficient and effective manner. Great care was taken to identify the desired outcomes being sought and how they would be measured. These included improving clinical results, reducing the length of stay, increasing patient and staff satisfaction, reducing variation from the guidelines for care, and improving resource management. Measurement tools were developed for the collection of future data. The innovation that had the greatest impact on the patients and staff was the introduction of a preadmission testing phase. During this preadmission visit, patients were assessed by members of the multidisciplinary treatment team. Nurse managers Nancy Jo Schmitz and Charlotte Busone agreed that "the pathway has reduced the frustration of spending many nursing hours to prepare a patient for surgery, only to find that the patient's procedure would be canceled due to an undetected medical or social condition." According to Joel Melnikoff, kinesiotherapist, "From a rehabilitation point of view, having the patient know what to expect really helps with having motivated patients [who are] able to perform their exercises."

The first patient was admitted on the pathway in March 1993. Since then we have had approximately fifty patients (at an average of about twenty per year) admitted to the pathway. A comparison of lengths of stay prior to the pathway to those after pathway implementation shows a decrease from 14.5 days (from the time of admission to acute care to the time of discharge to home or rehabilitation) to 8.1 days. Although patients perceived their care to be good to excellent prior to the establishment of the clinical pathway, patient satisfaction surveys administered postdischarge after the introduction of the pathway indicated an overall increase in the percentages of perceived excellence in physician care, nursing care, overall care, and discharge instructions. Membership in the Iroquois Consortium enabled the team to benchmark with community hospitals utilizing the same measurement tools.

The pathway is a living document, and as such it is continuously being reviewed and revised. The core committee remains in existence, and in addition to maintaining oversight of the total hip replacement clinical pathway, it is currently in the process of developing a total knee replacement pathway. A storyboard displaying the TQI tools used (that is, flowcharts and bar graphs), the steps taken to develop the pathway, and the results of pre- and postpathway data collection was created by the team and is used for information sharing both inside and outside the facility.

Author: Sara LaMarca graduated from St. John's Episcopal Hospital School of Nursing, Brooklyn, in 1966 and has worked in the VA health care system for seventeen years in various capacities. She has been a TQI consultant at the Stratton VA medical center for approximately seven years, with primary responsibility for support of surgical services. She is active in several process improvement teams and is currently working on expanding clinical pathway development throughout the medical center.

Reference
Scholtes, P. R. (1988). *The team handbook*. Madison, WI: Joiner Associates.

Chapter Thirteen

A Look at Team Dynamics, Training, Successes, and Pitfalls

Kenneth D. Flint, Judith A. Lerner, Evereteen Mayfield, and Kathryn K. St. Morris

The work of teams is recognized as the backbone of total quality improvement (TQI). The literature is replete with examples of well-constructed teams and instructions on how to use them to accomplish major improvements. As the Veterans Health Administration (VHA) began the planning and development of its TQI effort, it placed good teamwork on the same high plateau as leadership participation, regarding both as equally important. We developed special training for team members and had our consultants focus on team leaders and facilitators to ensure that all team members received ample attention in the early training sessions. But in spite of this recognition of the importance of teams and their needs, we found that in many places teamwork did not come easily or without problems.

Part of the problem VHA had with teams in the early part of the implementation related to issues that others have seen before—not timing the training to fit the circumstances or not having the right mix of individuals on a given team. But there were specific issues that arose during VHA's experience that were undoubtedly caused by some of the unique circumstances of hospital care or a large government bureaucracy.

First, patient care processes, especially those in a hospital, are cross-functional in nature and thus involve many different disciplines. As the target problem becomes larger in scope—which may occur when the chartering process leads to broad, vaguely defined areas assigned for evaluation—more and more disciplines must be involved in the change process. While other organizations may have encountered the issue of having many different disciplines represented on teams addressing a given problem, it is not a widely shared concern outside of health care. It is not the *number* of disciplines represented on health care TQI teams that causes problems, however; it is the *diversity* of these disciplines that may slow the team down, as interdisciplinary learning must occur among the different members. For instance, a cross-functional team evaluating the discharge process of a hospital service that treats recent amputees might require a physician, one or more nurses, clerical personnel from both inpatient and outpatient areas, possibly a representative from radiology, a social worker, and probably a staff member from the prosthetics division. In such teams the gaps in each member's knowledge about the activities of the others can be quite astounding. VHA not only anticipated this situation but actually looked forward to it, because the learning that would take place in such teams would create a solid foundation for future problem solving. We had no idea of the magnitude of the knowledge gaps our teams would have to fill in, however, nor of the time it would take for such diverse team members to become comfortably aware of one another's activities.

In addition, a second, somewhat more polarizing problem developed as a result of team diversity. Team members not only had widely varied duties but also widely varied backgrounds and education, and these differences did produce difficulties. The spectrum of personal experience among the members of a hospital TQI team may be quite broad. Some may have worked in their particular field for their entire career, while others may have limited experience in their field or in health care in general—or in any job. For example, a career employee from the prosthetics service who is trying to solve a problem in the ordering and delivery of prostheses may, on a TQI team, be asked to work with a ward clerk who is a recent high school graduate. Others on the team may also have vastly different experience and educational backgrounds, from those who have a doctoral degree to those who are still working on a bachelor's or master's degree. Again, such diversity and the exchange of information it would require was anticipated by VHA to be a positive force. What we did not anticipate, however, was the time commitment necessary for team members to bridge the gaps between their backgrounds and education before they could begin to function as a team. While these issues created mostly time delays, there were instances where the gaps seemed to be the root cause of problems that threatened to derail the team.

Others have stressed the need to involve physicians from the start (Godfrey, Berwick, & Roessner, 1992; Wakefield & Wakefield, 1993); the plan in VHA was to make a special effort to see that physicians were welcomed into the team atmosphere (see Chapter Seven). Most of the issues dealt with by other authors relate to physicians' not being hospital employees and how hospitals can attract them to become interested and involved. In VHA the situation is somewhat different, however, since the physicians on staff are in large measure also employees of the system. They face the same frustrations faced by all other VHA employees, and this would seem to lower any barriers to their involvement. But VHA physicians are just as busy as those in private practice, albeit in the hospital and not at some distance away in an office building. Thus, dealing with the physician staff in VHA posed some unique opportunities and problems, as it was crucial to secure their early involvement and to keep their attention during the time it took for teams to iron out the wrinkles and address the issues at hand. (Chapter Seven provides a detailed examination of the special needs and contributions of physicians in the TQI process.)

Systemwide Experiences

The thirty-eight hospitals involved in Phase I and Phase II of VHA's TQI implementation each chartered a number of teams within a few weeks of completing their process assessments. As we progressed through the implementation process, we became aware of the value of sharing information between sites on team activities. Information about what kinds of teams were formed at other hospitals and what kinds of members were appointed to them was seen as highly useful. Therefore, VHA's Office of Quality Management (OQM) and Quality Management Institute (QMI) decided to create a database to provide this type of information. A database was devised using VHA's national electronic communications system and housed at the QMI in Durham, North Carolina. Access to the database was through VHA's E-mail system, FORUM. The database was quite simple and included only basic information about the teams. Each facility was encouraged to access the database regularly and to enter information on their teams for use throughout the system. Individuals could make entries about their team's assigned topic and its membership and include other narrative information at any time; most entries were made soon after a team was chartered and were later updated by hospital staff.

In mid-1995, when the database was about two years old, the information entered by the thirty-eight hospitals participating in Phase I and Phase II was extracted from the database and analyzed. Not all hospitals had used the database capability; twenty-six of the thirty-eight facilities had made multiple entries over time. A total of 317 teams were identified from the electronic database; these teams had been established since early 1992. Facility participation in the database varied from a single team entry for two facilities to more than twenty by five facilities. Why some facilities did not participate in the database is not known; they may not have wished to have the information on their activities available for others to see and review. Some of the other twelve facilities were individually contacted and asked for a list of their teams and topics to complete the database information for Phases I and II. Six of these responded and submitted a list of their teams and topics for inclusion.

Analysis of the team data included determining the number of cases reported by each facility, arranging the topics addressed by the teams into major groupings, and further categorizing the topics according to the distinctive type of problem each team evaluated. For this last effort, the topics were assigned to categories by two different observers, using a set of decision-making rules. The categories and rules were as follows:

1. *Purely administrative:* the process being examined is not related to any diagnostic or treatment-related activity (for example, reducing the paperwork in an administrative department).
2. *Administrative with direct patient care implications:* The process is mostly of an administrative nature, but it directly affects patient

care in some way (for example, a system for ensuring that abnormal test results are brought to the attention of the responsible physician).

3. *Clinical with a significant administrative component:* The process directly relates to patient care issues but involves administrative processes as well (for example, designing a palliative care unit).

4. *Purely clinical activity:* The process falls entirely within the realm of one or more clinical departments, and the issue relates entirely to direct patient care processes such as diagnosis or treatment (for example, improving diabetic foot care).

The combined database for Phase I and II hospitals contained information on 455 teams and the topics they were assigned to study and correct. Of these, 27 percent were purely administrative in nature, 49 percent were administrative with some direct clinical impact, 16 percent were clinical with an administrative component, and only 8 percent were purely clinical. Within those categories, the most common topics teams were assigned to improve were as follows:

1. *Administrative*
   Improve movement of paperwork (such as claims)
2. *Administrative with clinical impact*
   Improve scheduling
   Improve patient movement
   Improve admission or discharge processes
3. *Clinical with administrative component*
   Improve triage of clinic patients
   Improve response to patient complaints
4. *Purely clinical*
   Improve a diagnostic process
   Improve a treatment process

On average, each facility chartered three teams in the first wave and followed with additional teams within four to six months. The first teams chartered at each facility were assigned problems determined by the assessment process to be of a fairly high priority; fairly soon, however, issues that had not shown up high on the assessments were assigned to TQI teams. The most common initial team topics at the thirty-eight Phase I and Phase II facilities were as follows, in order of frequency (shown in parentheses):

1. Surgery cancellations (21)
2. Discharge planning (20)
3. Admissions processing (20)
4. Medical record retrieval (16)
5. Patient transportation (13)

The following were the most frequent topics addressed by the second wave of team chartering:

1. Intradepartmental issues
2. The TQI process
3. Public relations
4. Shelter for the homeless
5. Food quality

The relationship between the team topics and the facility's initial assessment of high-priority items disappears between the first and second wave of team formation, a period usually of less than six months.

The teams originally chartered were called process action teams (PATs). These teams were expected to describe the status of the function or process they were evaluating and gather a body of facts to outline its strengths and weaknesses. Members of such teams were expected to bring a detached objectivity to their work; they were not chosen for their expertise in the subject matter. As the first explorers of the circumstances, they were expected to present a clear definition of the problem but not to fix anything. The chartering body—the quality leadership team (QLT)—intended to take the work of the PATs and use it to determine the need for additional teams of different types and constituencies to address possible solutions to the problem.

Process improvement teams (PITs) were then chartered to take the first steps of the PAT and use TQI tools and methods to develop a thorough understanding of the process and the probable root causes of the problems it presented. Members of these teams were chosen because of their knowledge of the process. These teams were assigned to work on chronic, multidisciplinary issues and to find ways of making some improvement—usually the target goal was 10 to 15 percent—in the process. In fact, over 65 percent of the initial teams chartered were asked to both *assess* and *correct* the process they were studying. Examples of such teams were the discharge medication turnaround team and the recharging medical records team at the VA hospital in San Diego. In many instances, the teams were asked to identify the process improvement steps they thought would be most likely to succeed and then make recommendations to the QLT concerning how to implement them.

As the master trainers and the staff at the VA hospitals became more comfortable with the TQI process, they began to use the team concept to address issues and needs other than those identified in the assessment process. Teams were created to help with the planning and design of major new efforts, including the installation of a new computer system and the addition of a new building annex. In this regard, TQI principles were used not to *fix* identified problems but to *prevent* problems from developing in the future. This represents a natural progression of the use of the philosophy and tools of quality improvement, a progression that was evident at some of the hospitals even at an early stage in the national implementation. Often the best members for design teams were individuals with some political muscle, particular planning skills, or resource ownership.

The great majority of the issues addressed by TQI teams in the Phase I and Phase II hospitals were predominantly administrative. Although these administrative processes could honestly be said to support and assist in the clinical care of patients, the bulk of the process steps were of a strictly administrative nature and did not require any clinical input or skill to understand or to suggest improvements. The choice of such topics was driven, in most instances, by the hospital assessment process. Physician involvement was more difficult to obtain and maintain on administratively focused teams, and several hospitals needed to focus attention on this issue.

Team Experiences

Team Chartering

A key part of the TQI process is the proper use of teams to assess issues and find solutions to problems. There is more hard work than magic in the team process, and an important aspect of accomplishing team goals is understanding exactly what is expected. The mechanism for accomplishing that understanding is the team charter.

Normally the charter should set the stage for the work and the activities of the team. It is a bridge between the part of the organization responsible for strategy and the members of the TQI teams. The communication provided by the charter may arguably be the single most important part of a team's history; the charter is both a communication tool and a road map that will help the team reach its goal.

A properly constructed charter will include several salient and critical items concerning the target of the team's efforts, the boundaries of the organization's expectations, the resources available to the team to accomplish its goal, and the time line for the activity. The following are important items that should be clearly defined in every team charter:

- The process to be addressed by the team
- The limits, or boundaries, of the scope of the team's activities
- The process owner (the person with the authority or resources to change the process under study)
- The resources available to the team during the course of its work
- The expected time line for the work
- The level of authority held by the team
- The level of improvement anticipated

Preliminary studies by VHA's Western Region Special Studies Group and the staff of the Long Beach regional medical education center (RMEC) have shown that 38 percent of the variation in team outcomes was related to three specific causes: team charters, length of time the team was in place, and the commitment of the appropriate manager (often the service or department chief). Of these three, the most significant predictor of good outcomes was a written charter for the team.

Chartering of teams that will address issues involving critical success factors for the entire organization should be done at the very top of the organization. In the early phases of the TQI implementation at most VA hospitals, there was a top-level management team—either a QLT or a steering committee—responsible for organizational assessment, prioritization of the areas identified as needing improvement, and establishment and chartering of appropriate teams. Under the plan conceived by the consultants and endorsed by VHA, the proper sequence of events following assessment and prioritization was as follows:

1. The QLT develops a team charter.
2. The QLT chooses employees to form a team.
3. The team members receive the necessary training to do their task.
4. The team does the assigned review.
5. The team reports its findings and actions to the QLT.

In fact, this sequence was not followed in many cases, and as a result the process developed some unique problems and solutions.

An early problem, noted by nearly every master trainer and present in virtually every hospital, related to team charters that were unfocused, vague, or too broad for the teams to grasp or understand. This phenomenon was known as the "solve world hunger" charter; the concept or issue assigned to the team was of such size and complexity that it was impossible for the team to even begin to understand exactly what they were being asked to do.

When closely examined, this problem itself was complex and multifaceted. At first blush it appeared that the QLTs were simply not defining the issues at hand for the teams. But a closer examination by several master trainers who were trying to help facilities understand their tasks better disclosed at least two types of problems in the vagueness of such charters. First, there was the easily recognized issue of the too-large scope of the charter. Statements of the problem were often of enormous width, such as "Fix Medical Records," "Improve Patient Transport," or "Fix Discharge Planning." Some of the teams were not even enjoined to "fix" anything but had charters centered on "Employee Education" or "Patient Satisfaction." Clearly the team assigned one of these topics will need much more guidance before embarking on its mission.

The team faced with "Employee Education" at the Columbus, Ohio, outpatient clinic wrestled with the question of whether they should focus their time and energy on the type and breadth of educational offerings at the facility or on whether what was currently offered actually accomplished the mandatory training requirements. They chose the second option and made their findings relevant to the penetration of existing training into the workforce.

The second type of vague chartering problem noted by the master trainers related to the lack of specific key information, such as who the presumed process owner was and whether that process owner was informed about or aware of the team's activities. Other items that were frequently covered vaguely or skimpily—or not at all—were such details as the amount of time the QLT was allowing the team to do its work or to what extent the team could call for resources such as data collection or analysis to assist it in accomplishing its task.

Also, the presumption that the QLTs simply needed to give a little more attention to this chartering issue was found to understate the needs of the facilities. As many as half of the QLTs seen by the master trainers who were interviewed did not actually prepare the charters themselves. The responsibility for developing the charter, and sometimes for transmitting it to the team, was delegated to the executive assistant for TQI. Since the QLTs were uninvolved in developing the charters, they could not answer various questions raised by the teams; they also did not learn anything from their contact with the teams, since they lacked a basic understanding of the teams' assigned tasks.

The QLTs' abdication of their responsibility to write clear charters was traced to their ignorance of the process and of the importance of a properly drafted charter. Even in those facilities where the TQI consultant had stressed the critical nature of the charter and its effect on the function and success of TQI teams, the QLTs rarely had any training in drafting team charters or any close oversight by the consultant. As a consequence, the members of the QLT were both uncomfortable with the chartering process and unaware that they needed to find out more about it.

For these facilities, the lesson learned was obvious: the QLT needed to be educated about the importance of chartering teams properly and adequately trained in the chartering process. In the absence of such training, most of the facilities that were having trouble with vague or "world hunger" charters developed other means of answering the questions of team members. Several hospitals allowed their teams to renegotiate their charter with the QLT after they had studied it and developed preliminary goals. These goals were then hashed out with the QLT until the targeted issue was one the QLT thought was important and the team felt was sufficiently specific and clear that they could make some headway in addressing it. No one thought the right answer to this problem was simply to obtain proper training for the executive assistant for TQI and leave the QLT out of the chartering process. In general, problems with lack of clarity, identifying process owners, setting boundaries, and designating resources were addressed by the negotiation method.

Another key action taken by several of the hospitals was to assign a liaison or a mentor from the QLT to meet with the team or the team leader regularly and provide guidance about the QLT's goals. In virtually every one of these instances the communication was immediately two-way. The resulting learning experience on the part of the QLT, both about the targeted issues and about the need for clarity in charters, is a good example of continuous improvement; this was noted both by members of the QLT and by the various teams.

Finally, a common theme, mentioned by two-thirds of the master trainers interviewed, was the limitations of the requirement to simply recommend changes to the QLT rather than actively pursue them. Many thought this was likely a byproduct of the chartering process and commented on the need to truly empower team members to *make* necessary changes rather than to simply pass a set of recommendations on to the "higher-ups." That practice of passing responsibility upward has been the modus operandi of VHA for years; while it protects rank-and-file employees from the consequences of any decision that goes awry, it also deprives them of the ability to make the improvements they know will enhance the efficiency or quality of their work process.

The chartering process is important for a variety of reasons and should not be taken lightly. VA hospitals are fortunate to have diligent employees who consistently ask for help and guidance when they need it. We are also fortunate to have attentive and innovative QLT members, who recognize needed improvements and, in the course of the TQI implementation, have used several different ways to bring them about. Lastly, the system is fortunate to have its dedicated corps of master trainers, who throughout the implementation have been available and willing to help make changes in operating processes, as long as it moved their facilities forward toward continuous improvement.

Team Composition

The composition of TQI teams is an important issue for the QLT or chartering body. If the members are not chosen carefully, there may be a critical talent or capability missing from the team. This can be a particular problem when chartering a team to deal with an issue that is so well focused and limited that all the team members come from the same background or process area. One hospital created a team to address one such limited issue and drew all the team members from shift employees familiar with the problem and the root issues. Unfortunately, these employees rotated to night or evening shifts frequently enough that scheduling team meetings was difficult; even when they were all working the day shift it was hard to gather enough members of the team to carry out its business. This team had to be dissolved.

The experience of a diverse team at the Fayetteville, North Carolina, VA hospital was completely different. Audits of medical records found a noncompliance rate at the hospital of 10 to 30 percent in meeting the requirement that routine consultations be completed within forty-eight hours of the time the order for them is written. A multidisciplinary team was chartered, composed of the relevant senior physicians, the chief of staff, the chief of nursing, and some administrative personnel, including the chiefs of ward administration, information resources, and medical administration. This team evaluated the problem, reviewed several alternatives, and created a capability in the decentralized hospital computer program (DHCP) for entry, notification, and follow-up of routine consultations. Training for the physician, nursing, and administrative staffs was provided, and subsequent audits found virtually no instances of noncompliance. Clearly, the success of this team was rooted in the team membership; the major process owners were part of the team, and the resources necessary to solve the problem were controlled by the members of the team.

Team Training

Training often posed an unexpected problem for the TQI teams. One unanticipated problem arose from the fact that many employees had never before experienced working in teams or in such an intense group activity. The pilot facilities found that employees needed training in basic team member and group skills before beginning a TQI project. In retrospect, the teams that functioned best seemed to be the ones that received some orientation in this area—usually involving an examination of team member roles and a brief introduction to the tools of team-based problem solving—and were left to do their business; detailed training in the use of specific TQI tools was scheduled by the team facilitator or mentor when the need arose. This "just-in-time" training seemed to meet everybody's needs: the trainer was not frustrated by having to repeat training, and teams were able to focus their time and effort on what was needed at the time. This type of training was provided by the master trainers as the need arose; occasionally training could be provided to a team by one of its members, as was the case at the Boise VA hospital, where the associate chief of staff for ambulatory care was both a team member and a trainer for a team investigating misdirected laboratory specimens.

Another important training issue in the pilot hospitals was the recognized necessity for team facilitators. In those hospitals with a high degree of TQI activity and many chartered teams, the need for team facilitators was often large. The facilitator's role in assisting with team training is critical to a TQI team's success. At the Hines VA hospital in Chicago, one of the early teams involved members of the dietetic department—two registered dietitians and five food service workers trying to improve the timeliness of the delivery of evening supplements to the hospital wards. None of the team members had experience or training in the TQI process. The hospital arranged for an experienced TQI facilitator to provide leadership and just-in-time training to the team. They worked at the improvement process for eight months and finally developed improvements that resulted in reduced personnel costs, reduced food wastage, and improved customer (patient and ward nurse) satisfaction. The San Diego hospital arranged to have more than twenty of its employees trained in the facilitation of a variety of support functions, from straightforward teamwork facilitation by process improvement teams to facilitating management retreats.

One of the biggest lessons learned by both the individual hospitals and by systemwide TQI practitioners was that teams needed ongoing training in a variety of topic areas, ranging from systematic problem solving to data collection and analysis to report writing. As one of the master trainers put it, "training is forever." The recognition of this need was not entirely new to those planning the implementation. A detailed education and training plan had already been created before the first site officially began its involvement with TQI. The levels of training required and the amount of training delivered varied quite a bit across the thirty-eight Phase I and Phase II sites. (A more detailed description of the training plan and its implementation is presented in Chapter Six.)

Team Communication

Communication became a hot topic at some time in the life of nearly every team. As one wag said, "The biggest myth about communication is that it happened." In spite of the best intentions, information about what was happening in a team and about its progress often did not get into the right hands at the right time. At other times, miscommunication or a breakdown in communication created barriers to proper team functioning; these circumstances called for early recognition and prompt action to relieve the problem before the team lost momentum.

A retrospective evaluation of team communication at the various hospitals revealed two distinct types of miscommunication. The first type was miscommunication within a team. One form of this was squabbling or bickering between team members from different disciplines. Participants in TQI must learn and adhere to the rules of conduct for TQI team members; otherwise, certain team members may continually upset the flow of the conversation by interjecting their opinions about the beliefs and motivations of members from other disciplines. Often such individuals bring to their team experience a certain amount of "baggage" from past relationships with members of particular disciplines; such issues may require some airing before the team can move on. The best remedy for this type of miscommunication is to invoke the rules of team conduct and to review the training on the role of teams and team members in the TQI process (to remind team members of why they are there).

Another form of intrateam miscommunication, especially prevalent in teams containing individuals from many different disciplines, was the habitual use of jargon or arcane vocabularies not familiar to other team members. In some cases this led to the development of a "team within a team"—and the subsequent disenfranchisement of the other members. The group leader and facilitator need to be aware of the danger of allowing lengthy "explanations" by some members that monopolize the team's time.

Occasionally, a VHA team ran into difficulties when an employee and his or her supervisor were both on the same team. This situation is not necessarily unproductive, but in a few instances it caused employees to fail to speak up for fear of contradicting their supervisor. When both an employee and his or her supervisor are an important source of information about the process under evaluation—or when they are both, to some degree, process owners—their presence together on the team is important. Special attention needs to be paid to this issue by the team leader and team facilitator.

The second major communication difficulty faced by VHA teams was keeping those who were not part of a given team aware of the team's progress and thinking about the process the team was evaluating. There were some instances in which a team's failure to adequately communicate their progress to an important outside individual—often a manager or supervisor who also happened to be a significant process owner—directly led to the team's proposed remedies being delayed or not employed at all. Those hospitals where particular attention was paid to communicating team activities (especially for those teams where the process owners were involved) had a higher rate of success and sustained greater interest in the TQI effort across the facility. The Lexington hospital's practice of having the QLT meet with the teams and process owners at the beginning of each team's activities worked well and was adopted at other sites as well.

Communication with individuals or departments outside the team seemed to be particularly difficult in cases where the process changes being considered crossed major turf lines in the hospital. In one instance, a team was unable to obtain the data it needed to assess a process because the owner of that process simply refused to share the data. Intervention from the QLT was necessary to ensure that the data was available for the team to review.

In another instance of poor communication, a team studying ways of improving the movement of paperwork throughout their facility recommended that the hospital install pneumatic tubes to connect its various services. The plan required substantial physical modifications to the hospital building. The team's recommendations were brought to the QLT at virtually the same time that the hospital leadership decided to cease all new construction in the inpatient area in favor of upgrading the ambulatory care areas. The team had operated in isolation from the realities and new strategic goals of the hospital.

There were some examples of communication between teams and the hospital leadership that worked well and had a far-reaching impact. One VA hospital routinely required TQI team members to give presentations on their work to the QLT. The first time one kitchen aide stood in front of the hospital director to make his report, his hands were trembling and the paper he was holding shook visibly. The next time he appeared for a presentation, however, he was calm, articulate, and in complete control of himself and his material. This kind of communication experience as a part of the team function repeatedly served as a source of personal and professional growth for many staff.

Team Functionality

Team functionality often depended on the ability of the team leader or facilitator to solve rather mundane problems. Some teams had difficulty meeting because of scheduling conflicts between members. Occasionally the greatest need was for team training for all members so that they would know what was expected of them. In a few instances the team members were eager to progress to problem solving before the issue was clear or before sufficient information had been collected.

In some cases the process data uncovered by a team came as a complete surprise to the team members. One example was a team that was trying to improve the availability of patients' medical records in the triage area of its facility's outpatient clinic. The team had ample data indicating that charts were available to the triage physician only about 8 percent of the time. The team was charged with investigating "Is the chart always available, and if not, why not?" Team members were drawn from both suppliers and customers of the process of delivering medical records to the triage area. The team had several ideas about the *probable* causes of the problem, but they decided to create a list of the myriad *possible* causes anyway. They then collected specific information relating to each of these causes and ranked the items by frequency. To their surprise, the most common reason for no chart being sent to the triage area was that no request was ever made for it. This single issue, which was not anticipated by the team members, accounted for fully 25 percent of the instances where no chart arrived in triage.

Sometimes a team's solution to a problem creates new problems elsewhere. This happened at the Oklahoma City VA hospital. A TQI team composed entirely of emergency room nurses there "solved" the problem of transferred patients having to wait long periods before they were screened by physicians and admitted to a ward. The nurses' "solution" was to directly divert the transferred patients to the wards. Unfortunately, the ward physicians and nurses were unaware of this change in procedure, and one patient was sent to a ward at 4:00 P.M. but not seen by a physician until after midnight, by which time he had suffered complications. The previous "solution" was revisited, this time with a team containing players from all involved departments. A new process was developed that met the emergency room's need to not have its space tied up for long periods by transferred patients and the receiving ward's need to be aware of the existence and status of newly admitted patients. A major lesson learned here was that solutions crafted by an incomplete group of stakeholders can lead to unexpected and adverse results.

Lessons Learned

A wide variety of team experiences occurred in the thirty-eight Phase I and Phase II hospitals. As teams learned from their own successes and failures, the master trainers and TQI oversight committees realized they could also learn from each other. The TQI teams database was created for that purpose, and on several occasions team stories were gleaned from the sites or the database to serve educational purposes. Some of those stories and the lessons learned from them are described below:

1. At the Little Rock VA hospital, personnel in the clinical laboratory noted that some patients' identification bracelets were difficult—almost impossible—to read. Recognizing the risk to patients from this hazard, the laboratory began accumulating data about the problem. Technicians were given a set of readability criteria, which they applied to the bracelets on all patients presenting to the laboratory for testing. Thirty percent of the identification bracelets they examined were classifiable as unreadable. This information was transmitted to the department responsible for making the bracelets, medical administration; they responded by purchasing a new type of bracelet with virtually indelible printing.

Although there was no baseline data about errors due to unreadable bracelets, the indisputable benefits of the reduced likelihood of erroneous drug administration or transfusion errors were significant. These benefits demonstrate what can result from a self-generated team activity in a single department.

2. The social work service at the Hines VA hospital in Chicago perceived an unnecessary paperwork burden in the facility's requirement that case data be entered on case registry forms by social work staff and then later entered into the DHCP by clerical personnel. They determined that the work load averaged about two thousand forms per month and the average error rate was 5 to 6 percent (100 to 120 rejected code sheet entries each month). The team recommended that social work staff should make entries directly into the DHCP. Training and additional terminals were obtained, and the changeover was made. A direct improvement was noted in the accuracy of the data entered into the DHCP (only a 0.8 percent error rate), and side benefits included increased cler-

ical staff time for other duties and increased staff proficiency in using other computer software packages. Lessons learned included the gaining of side benefits when a primary process is improved.

3.   At the Boise VA hospital, two patients had abnormal chest radiographs that could have led to early diagnosis and treatment, but they were not diagnosed until later in the course of their disease. Review of hospital activity indicated that each month, ten to twelve abnormal radiographs were not promptly brought to the attention of the responsible physician. The facility created a team of involved clinicians who developed a flowchart of the process, a cause-and-effect diagram that identified a wide variety of potential reasons, and collected data over three months. They used the information they gathered to construct a solution using the DHCP to record, track, and provide follow-up for all abnormal chest films. The number of cases not promptly identified fell to the level of isolated events. The lesson learned was that even processes that seem simple are often much more complex than is apparent from first evaluation.

4.   Review of the occurrence screening data at the VA hospital in Kansas City disclosed that the rate of nosocomial pneumonia was higher on some nursing units than on others. A team of clinicians from nursing, respiratory care, pulmonary medicine, surgery, and other services reviewed the available data and discovered that higher rates of nosocomial pneumonia occurred among patients who received respiratory therapy from nursing staff rather than from respiratory therapists. Their solution involved shifting responsibility for respiratory therapy from nursing to respiratory care and developing a computer-based work assessment system. The reorganization took several months because of the need to transfer personnel from nursing to respiratory care and recruit new respiratory therapists. Nurses were pleased with the change in responsibility, and respiratory care was happy with the new system and their ability to provide care to all patients needing it. The nosocomial pneumonia rate decreased by more than 50 percent. Lessons learned included that clinicians can employ TQI tools to solve clinical problems and directly improve care.

5.   The Oklahoma City VA hospital admitted a patient with a diabetic foot ulcer; the patient had been seen a week before in the clinic, but the ulcer was not detected. Recognizing that foot ulcers

are the most common reason for hospitalization in diabetics and that regular foot care can reduce their incidence, hospital staff reviewed the medical records of one hundred diabetic patients and discovered that only 10 percent of them passed American Diabetic Association (ADA) guidelines for laboratory and physical examinations, including foot examinations. A team of clinicians reviewed the ADA guidelines and developed a series of recommendations, including monitoring the quality of care; educating patients, nurses, and physicians on proper diabetic foot care; and creating a data collection system to monitor compliance with ADA guidelines for examinations. One year after initiating the changes, more than 90 percent of these examinations met the ADA guidelines, and the number of diabetics admitted for foot ulcers decreased by 50 percent. Lessons learned included that clinical processes can be significantly improved by the introduction of subject matter expertise in the process design.

6.   The Albany VA hospital's hospital-based home care (HBHC) program was responsible for collecting laboratory specimens from patients in their homes. To do so, HBHC nurses needed certain supplies, which were scattered about the hospital. Laboratory staff were asked to accompany HBHC nurses on their home visits, and they quickly discovered that laboratory policies and practices caused difficulty for the HBHC program. Specifically, widely dispersed specimen containers and collection methods designed for inpatient use were wasting the nursing staff's time. The multidisciplinary team from the two departments addressed each of these issues and produced a set of collection and transport criteria for HBHC specimens that fit the needs of the program without compromising laboratory standards. They also created an "HBHC lab bag" containing all the needed supplies; stocking and refilling of the bag was the responsibility of the laboratory staff as a service to their customers, the HBHC nurses. A major lesson learned here was that departments do not always know the needs of their customers and that they are able to quickly see how to improve their processes once they walk through them with their customers.

In each of these stories, a team of interested employees addressed a key process that was not running smoothly. They used simple TQI tools, made sometimes startling discoveries about root causes, and were able to make significant improvements. Even clinicians became involved and made substantive changes in their processes. The work of TQI teams, especially cross-functional teams, developed credibility in each of these hospitals as a result.

The great importance of teams in implementing TQI was recognized by VHA in the course of its TQI pilot program. This recognition was reflected in the fact that the steering committees were renamed quality leadership *teams* at most hospitals and in the realization that they, too, needed team training. The team concept should have been initially modeled by the "core four," but it became apparent during Phase I that many of these groups did not function like teams; VHA recognized that deficiency and made significant improvements in Phase II.

References

Godfrey, A. B., Berwick, D. M., & Roessner, J. (1992, April). Can quality management really work in health care? *Quality Progress*, pp. 23–27.

Wakefield, D. S., & Wakefield, B. J. (1993, March). Overcoming the barriers to implementation of TQM/CQI in hospitals: Myths and realities. *Quality Review Bulletin*, pp. 83–88.

Chapter Fourteen

A Regional Perspective

*John C. Lammers, Stuart C. Gilman,
and Kenneth J. Clark*

The western region of the Veterans Health Administration (VHA)
administered from eighteen to thirty-six VA facilities between 1987
and 1995, when it was superseded by a major structural reorganization. During this period, the western region was recognized for
leadership in total quality improvement (TQI). Its employees
spoke at national meetings, such as the National Forum for Quality Improvement in Health Care and meetings of the American
Public Health Association. Representatives from the western region also held membership on many national planning committees such as the national TQI Evaluation Committee. Moreover,
the western region's medical centers were disproportionately represented in the early applications to participate in VHA's national
TQI implementation effort. The region has also been the home of
one of the few published studies of TQI in large multisite organizations (Lammers, Cretin, Gilman, & Calingo, forthcoming).

This chapter explores some reasons for TQI activity in the western region (hereafter called simply the "region"). We will show that
TQI activity in the region's facilities is attributable to multiple factors, including leadership, training, and incentives. First, we offer
a very brief history of TQI in the region. Second, we discuss penetration of TQI into the region's facilities and summarize the findings of region-sponsored research. Third, we explore how the
region's influence was experienced at the local level. Finally, we
discuss how this experience may be generalized to other large or-

ganizations attempting quality improvement efforts at multiple sites, and we comment on the long-term impact of the TQI effort in the region.

A Brief History of TQI in the Western Region

The first interest in TQI in the region was noted in 1988, when several physicians and managers, participating in a major region committee called the Regional Planning Board began conversations about the quality improvement methods of Deming, Juran, and others. These individuals convinced the regional director to support their travel to several sites to study the implementation of what was then called total quality management (TQM). In March 1989, this delegation visited Florida Power and Light; Alliant Health in Louisville, Kentucky; and the West Paces Ferry Hospital of Hospital Corporation of America. Upon their return these individuals enthusiastically reported their belief in the new management methods to the regional director. The director supported disseminating TQM theory within the region, and he arranged for the region's (then) eighteen facility executives to receive a copy of Mary Walton's book *The Deming Management Method* (1986). In September 1989, the director also developed a small health policy section (the Western Region Special Studies Group) in the regional office.

During 1990, the region was expanded to encompass thirty-six facilities in the western half of the United States, from Montana to New Mexico on its eastern border to Alaska and Hawaii on its western border. In December 1990, the authors and Russell Tyler met to discuss both their mutual interest in TQM and how to foster awareness of TQM among VA facility directors. This informal group suggested to the new regional director that a formal TQM advisory group would be of value to the region. Such a group would advise the regional director on TQM training issues and on the use of small grants to foster TQM, and it would serve as a TQM education and information resource for the region's facilities. The director endorsed the establishment of a TQI steering committee for the western region and expanded its membership to fully represent the region. (The name change from TQM to TQI coincided with the emphasis from the central office favoring the latter.)

Implementing TQI in the Western Region, 1991 to 1995

The material in this section is drawn from the minutes of steering committee meetings, from archived documents, and from results of surveys conducted annually from 1991 to 1995 (refined and expanded each year). Some of this material has been presented at professional meetings, published, or accepted for publication. The TQI steering committee first sought to develop an awareness training program for executives of western region facilities. A needs assessment was conducted by surveying the region's thirty-six executives, and they were prepared for a day-long TQI awareness program to be held in July 1991. As of May 1991, eighty percent of these executives indicated in a survey that they were "extremely interested in continuous quality improvement." Seventy-two percent of them had already begun TQI activities, and 69 percent had formed quality councils. However, only two of the thirty-six facilities had a quality council actively overseeing trained multidisciplinary teams using statistical methods—the strict definition of a TQI implementation. This suggested to the committee that the facilities in the region wished to be categorized as "doing" TQI (perhaps because of peer pressure), but few had the full complement of time, financial resources, and commitment to achieve such programs. Such a discrepancy between stated goals and objective evidence of action led to an attempt in subsequent surveys to discriminate between mere claims of implementation and actual evidence of it.

Based on its findings, the committee focused its training efforts on the following underlying principles of TQI:

- Acceptance of responsibility by top management to continuously improve customer satisfaction
- Commitment from every level of the organization to meeting the needs and expectations of internal and external customers
- Focused use of organizational resources to meet organizational goals
- Delegation of authority for ensuring quality in daily work to employees at all levels of the organization
- Objective use of empirical data to guide decisions

- A structured system of rewards and recognition
- Use of teams of workers to solve problems and improve work processes
- Systematic, organization-wide training in the use of tools for group decision making, including flowcharts, Pareto diagrams, run charts, histograms, and cause-and-effect diagrams [adapted from Lammers, Cretin, Gilman, & Calingo, forthcoming; Marszalek-Gaucher & Coffey, 1990; Berwick, Godfrey, & Roessner, 1990; Imai, 1986]

The June 1991 awareness training event featured both an experienced physician executive from the Department of Defense and a consultant from a firm that had played a prominent role in the National Demonstration Project (Berwick, Godfrey, & Roessner, 1990). The steering committee reinforced the training event with a monthly newsletter, *The TQI Club Journal,* that reprinted a scholarly article on TQI along with a page of commentary by a member of the committee.

At that time, VHA's national TQI effort was still being designed, and little understanding existed at the local level on how to select from the large number of TQI consultants advertising their services to region facilities. The May 1991 survey showed that twelve facilities had used nine different consultants. The steering committee compiled and disseminated an annotated list of consultants, detailing the length of time they had been active with TQI, their experience using TQI in health care, their experience with VA facilities, and other information.

Between May 1991 and December 1992, the steering committee also oversaw the distribution of $264,417 in TQI grants. The regional director had approved $300,000, to be competitively awarded to region facilities that could demonstrate how the funds would be beneficial to their TQI effort. An average grant of $24,038 was provided to eleven facilities (out of twenty-six applicants) in the first funding cycle. It was expected that this external source of funds would serve several purposes. First, it allowed committed executives to demonstrate to their staff that there were benefits to pursuing total quality. At the same time, it allowed committed staff the opportunity to prove to their employees that rewards were available for pursuing total quality. Lastly, at a time when the national TQI effort was still nascent, the grants provided resources for early regional total quality efforts.

In December 1992, the second western region TQI survey showed some important changes. This survey, which targeted the executive assistants for TQI, found that thirty-five of the thirty-six facilities reported that they were carrying out TQI. Eighty-six percent of the facilities reported having a quality council or similar TQI oversight body in place, and 37 percent reported having provided TQI awareness training for 50 to 100 percent of their workforce. Eighty percent of the region's facilities reported using a consultant to help their implementation effort, and the total number of consultants used had grown. At least twenty different sources of external TQI consulting were reported, with 75 percent of the facilities reporting that they were either satisfied or extremely satisfied with the consultants' work. The 1992 TQI survey also asked about the adequacy of organizational resources for external consultants (from the VHA central office, region headquarters, and VHA training sources); only 42 percent of the respondents believed that these resources were adequate. Thus, facilities indicated continued interest in using external consultants but a lack of adequate resources for that purpose.

Also in 1992, the annual survey was modified to collect more specific data regarding teams. Among the principles for successful TQI implementation adopted by the region was the idea that process action teams are one of the few *moving parts* of total quality improvement. Much effort is focused on changing organizational cultures and on training to enable teams to be successful. Therefore, the survey was expanded to include not only quality coordinators and executive assistants for TQI but team leaders as well. Analyses of the region's team data have been reported elsewhere (Lammers & Gilman, 1993; Lammers, Gilman, & Calingo, 1993; Lammers & Gilman, 1994a, 1994b; Lammers, Cretin, Gilman, & Calingo, forthcoming; Lammers, Yudelson, & Gilman, 1995); here we report highlights of these data that are relevant to implementing regionwide or systemwide change.

In December 1992, the region identified 107 process action teams at 72 percent of its facilities. Eighty-five percent of these teams were less than eight months old, and 66 percent had received some type of training. At this time, 45 percent of the leaders of these teams reported no difference in the quality of the process their team was chartered to improve; 53 percent observed an increase in quality; and 2 percent observed a decrease. During this period most of the teams were in the initial stages of quality improvement, primarily using brainstorming and flowcharting to study their assigned process. A small minority (fewer than 10 percent) reported using quantitative techniques, such as run or control charts.

Based on the region's continued interest in TQI and the commitment of its leadership, a second round of grants was offered in 1993. In this round, twenty-six proposals were received and twelve funded, at an average of $22,678. Projects that were funded ranged from general TQI training for quality councils to very specific support for improving clinical processes such as the use of metered-dose inhalers, home glucose monitoring, and the ordering, dispensing, and administering of medication.

In October 1993, the region sponsored yet another conference at which successful TQI efforts were showcased and discussed and the relationship of TQI to other organizational change efforts (such as systems thinking) was presented. Additionally, in November 1993, the region sponsored a conference entitled "Making the Transition from QA to TQI" to assist facilities in preparing for accreditation reviews.

By the time of the third TQI survey in the western region (in September 1993), 225 process action teams had been identified (112 new teams since the 1992 survey). Forty-two of these had already disbanded, their tasks complete. Also in 1993, the TQI survey instrument was expanded to measure management commitment and training activity at each facility and to evaluate the activities of quality councils and individual teams. Early efforts to identify team activities and measure team success depended upon surveys of team leaders. We asked them to assess the quality of their assigned process both before their team had begun its work and as of the date of the survey (see Lammers, Cretin, Gilman, & Calingo, forthcoming, for a more complete description of this approach). This allowed us to compare teams at various points in their life cycle, to identify characteristics that contributed to team success, and to develop facility-wide improvement profiles based on all the teams at each facility. Findings from several detailed analyses of the 1993 data are summarized below:

- No differences in quality improvement were found between western region facilities that had participated in different phases of the national TQI implementation (Lammers & Gilman, 1994b). This suggested that region facilities as a group might provide a different environment than other facilities in the country.

- Quality improvement was positively related to middle management (service chief) commitment to TQI principles, quality council guidance, the use of trained facilitators, and an experienced quality council (Lammers & Gilman, 1993). These observations suggest that training efforts are usefully focused upon middle management and that the quality council plays an important role in fostering improvement.

- Conceptions of the goal of TQI appeared to vary by level. For example, management and leadership have a strategic view of quality improvement, while physicians and other workers are likely to have a more practical and tactical view of improvement (Lammers, Cretin, Gilman, & Calingo, forthcoming). Thus systemwide change efforts may be more productive if they take into account the various interests and concerns of individuals working at different levels of the organization.

- The relationship between commitment to TQI principles and TQI budgeting was not obvious. Although the 1993 data demonstrated significant variations in the different hospitals' commitment to TQI and their TQI budgets, higher budgets did not always follow from strong commitment. This may be because some organizations chose not to set aside a separate TQI budget, but rather expected resources from all parts of the organization to be devoted to quality improvement activities (Lammers, Cretin, Gilman, & Calingo, forthcoming). The impact of TQI budgets also varied according to the size of the hospital (in 1993, region facilities ranged in size from stand-alone outpatient clinics to a hospital with 1,105 beds, and their budgets ranged from $2.9 million to $227.1 million). This fact raised difficult questions about the role of resources in improvement. It appeared that the level of improvement achieved was independent of TQI budget levels; but finances are notoriously difficult to track in VHA, and the actual cost of improvement activities in these facilities is unknown.

- Improvement results varied by team age. Very young teams (less than ninety days old) generally reported less improvement than teams between three months and one year old, but some teams over one year old reported a lack of improvement (Lammers, Yudelson, & Gilman, 1995). Combined with other evidence, this may suggest the importance of an experienced quality council and a long-term effort to sustain improvement projects, as well as a close review of projects that have not reported success after one year.

• Commitment among physicians was found to be significantly related both to the amount of training provided and to total perceived improvement. This finding reinforces the need to provide specific support and training to physicians if TQI efforts are to be successful (Lammers, Cretin, Gilman, & Calingo, forthcoming).

• The use of data analysis tools was more highly correlated with perceived improvement than was the use of group process tools. This suggests that teams that advance to the point of collecting data are more likely to be successful.

Data from the September 1994 survey have yet to be fully analyzed. The survey recorded eighty-one new teams at thirty-three responding medical centers. The 1994 data demonstrated that team leaders' reports of progress reflected the stage of the TQI cycle their team had attained. In other words, perceived improvement grew as teams moved from defining and organizing their project to analyzing the problem, identifying its causes, designing and implementing improvement activities, and finally monitoring outcomes (Lammers & Gilman, 1995).

Finally, the 1995 data, just collected and now being entered into VHA's national team database, has yielded information on sixty-six teams at work in the western region. These data will provide an opportunity to compare teams and centers across regions and to study differences in clinical and nonclinical teams. These analyses are presently under way.

Growth of western region TQI implementation is summarized in Table 14.1. While the data collected cannot claim to perfectly describe implementation in the region, they suggest several tentative conclusions. Facility commitment to TQI grew over the period 1991 to 1995, with quality councils being formed at all but one facility (which faced a union challenge to its TQI program), and mean perceived quality improvement has risen with experience.

Table 14.1. Summary Indicators of TQI Implementation in Thirty-Six Western Region Facilities.

Indicator	Year				
	1991	1992	1993	1994	1995
Facilities with quality councils	18	30	30	35	35
Total number of teams	n/a	107	225	190	66
Number of new teams	n/a	107	132	81	66
Percent reporting improvement*	n/a	53.0	55.0	58.1	86.4

*This item represents the percentage of team leaders who reported that quality had improved in the process their team was working on since the team had formed, regardless of the team's age. See the discussion above regarding the effect of team age.

There has also been a decline in the formation of process action teams. Several reasons may be given for this decline. First, while every effort has been made to ensure completeness of the data, each year's survey results are incomplete to some degree. For example, the 1995 data collection coincided with Joint Commission on Accreditation of Healthcare Organizations (JCAHO) accreditation activities, and those data are known to be incomplete for that reason. Second, overall enthusiasm for TQI has likely waned as other management innovations have gained ascendancy (such as reengineering and self-directed work groups). [Editor's note: These "innovations" are perfectly compatible with the philosophy of TQI.] Finally, some leveling of implementation activities is to be expected, as facilities' TQI programs become somewhat routine.

In mid-1994, the western region TQI steering committee determined that its mission of providing awareness training and information to encourage facility directors to pursue TQI had been accomplished. The committee disbanded, leaving the region's facilities to the national networks, which by that time had become quite well developed.

Benefits of High-Level Organizational Leadership

In addition to having committed, devoted people at all levels and facilities interested in TQI and willing to share in the work of developing it, the western region enjoyed several benefits specifically related to the involvement of its top leadership. First, two successive regional directors sustained a high commitment to TQI. The first director provided TQI information to each medical center and committed the region's special studies group to promoting quality improvement. When the region was expanded and a new director appointed, there was an expansion of the region's TQI commitment in the form of conferences and grants to medical centers. The new director not only provided continuity rather than disruption but also committed a wealth of resources specifically for TQI—well over $500,000 over two years—directly to the region's facilities.

Second, well-known, credible people were involved in planning the region's TQI effort. In addition, other local endeavors pursued by both directors as well as by physicians and managers involved in TQI brought added credibility to the effort. This assisted in deploying the TQI strategy legitimately and authentically throughout the region. The word was pushed out and down from the regional office in San Francisco. Eventually, as the data indicate, TQI knowledge did penetrate every site.

From the point of view of a medical center executive in the late 1980s and early 1990s, the competing factors of cost and quality were falling into sharp relief; cost reductions threatened program closure or reduced capability. VA facility managers had to balance the realities imposed by the prevailing prices and wages in their community against the directives handed down from VHA headquarters and the regional office in San Francisco. The stiff competition faced by many western region facilities required them to drive out inefficiencies and smooth their operations in order to increase patient satisfaction and improve outcomes. In particular, VHA managers faced stiff competition for recruitment. The TQI features of employee empowerment and improved climate became a way to improve employee satisfaction, and it gave VHA managers a competitive edge. After the disappointing JCAHO scores of the late 1980s, VHA managers became more cognizant of the competition they faced from other community health care facilities. This was a switch from the historically isolationist position of most VA medical centers. Increasingly, VHA executives studied private sector initiatives like TQI in an effort to maintain comparable state-of-the-art programs and operations.

The dilemma faced by many VHA executives was to create a sense of urgency for change in their institution. Executives found it difficult to obtain enthusiastic support from key management staff for large TQI expenditures, such as for outside consultants. This problem was made more difficult because literature on the benefits of TQI was not then readily available, as it increasingly is today. One of the principal benefits of the region's TQI program for individual facilities was that it provided an external funding source that was immune to opposition from constituents who regarded internal funding of TQI as little more than "robbing Peter to pay Paul." The task of bringing influential middle managers into a change process like TQI often depends upon the availability of such external resources. In such cases, the availability of western region funds may have been the single most important factor in convincing management staff to take the leap of faith necessary to support the arduous task of implementing TQI.

The availability of TQI survey data also helped medical center executives push implementation of TQI at their own institutions. The data not only helped individual medical centers learn from the TQI experience of other facilities but also created positive peer pressure to support TQI implementation, even when it did not provide conclusive evidence of its efficacy. Meeting at region-sponsored or supported programs, medical center executives had an opportunity to compare practices and observations about what appeared to work; some executives adopted or continued TQI programs simply so they would not appear to their peers to be behind the times.

Isolating the tangible benefits of TQI implementation is difficult at best, particularly when balanced against the considerable time, energy, effort, and funds required for that implementation. The chief benefit may be the provision of a structure and process for arriving at a logical resolution to the myriad problems facing health care organizations. For example, traditionally most VA hospitals (like most other health care organizations) have operated using a structure of standing committees, whose principal responsibility is to maintain current systems and operations. Problem solving is usually addressed through the use of problem-specific task forces composed of the people from the organization who are most familiar with the problem being addressed. Unfortunately, in many instances the traditional approach leads to unsatisfactory results. Task forces are often composed of the same individuals most responsible for maintaining the status quo, and their members are in many instances unfamiliar with tools, techniques, and processes that lead to successful problem solving. Hence, longstanding problems tend to be addressed only periodically, in an approach to problem solving that is episodic at best. Such an approach usually addresses the symptoms of a problem but rarely the underlying process. Moreover, topic-specific task forces can proliferate to the point where meaningful management is nearly impossible. This results in inadequate follow-through in the completion of the task forces' initiatives, leaving problems unsatisfactorily resolved and in some cases exacerbated through the efforts of the task force.

The TQI approach offers remedies to both these problems, and both remedies benefit from the kind of support provided by the region. First, TQI requires the type of organizational support and resources that the region provided to its facilities, making available the necessary technical training to develop effective problem-solving behavior in organization employees. This is where the region's support of specific process action team projects paid off. Second, the region's symbolic support for the TQI approach and the resources it provided to involve mid-level managers and physicians were instrumental in creating a quality council or other steering committee at each facility to strategically identify areas for improvement and to empower and then keep track of project action teams. This led to far more coordinated and therefore successful management of limited medical center resources.

As one experienced medical center executive put it, "I'm still committed to the structure [of TQI]. It gets things done, it helps me martial forces throughout the medical center. The quality council identifies the problems, empowers teams to solve them. The teams study and recommend changes. Teams aren't formed or assigned unless change is needed. They don't just go off and are never heard from again. A good example is the high number of patients we had out on passes . . . some were turning up out on the street. It was a public relations nightmare. A process action team, accountable to the quality council, solved the problem. The old committee system protected old routines. Process action teams implement change, and the quality council keeps track of them."

This example illustrates how the total organization can become involved in change, and it demonstrates the structural role of a quality council empowered by regional resources and support.

Conclusion

In early discussions about TQI, the interest group recognized four motivating forces that could prompt an organization to adopt TQI:

1. The desire to expand in a market
2. Competitive pressures from other organizations
3. Ethical standards (a desire to provide safe products or services that are consistent with customers' or clients' value systems)
4. Mandates from authorities (like government regulators or, in the case of hospitals, JCAHO) [adapted from Tyler, 1988]

In retrospect, we recognized a fifth force that compelled adoption of TQI in the western region—namely, peer pressure. Each of these forces played a role in establishing TQI in western region facilities, and each can be used to continue to involve hospitals in large systems like VHA. While market forces do not classically play a role in government hospitals, in an era of reform, VHA managers understand that they face competition with other local facilities for patients and resources. Also, the West particularly is the scene of intense competitive pressures for many health sector inputs such as nurses, physicians, and insurance dollars. In addition, the region's lower-than-expected accreditation scores of the late 1980s made public both ethical and regulatory pressures for reform. Finally, western region facility executives, in discussions among themselves and with colleagues in non-VA facilities, shared a desire to continuously improve the performance of their organizations. However, we acknowledge that while peer pressure may propel initial adoption, it cannot by itself sustain implementation over the long haul.

Moreover, each of the motivators listed above can become elements of enlightened system design: each is dependent upon other system elements, and each can be objectively measured. For example, population-based health care, begun in VHA sites like the Pilot Ambulatory Care Education Center at Sepulveda, California, takes into account the needs, size, and characteristics of a given market for ambulatory care. Using TQI principles and system- or regional-level support, the market can be measured and the facility designed to meet its needs. Second, the competitive pressures on facilities can also be measured and managed. Using TQI principles and approaches, system-level managers can listen and respond to medical center executives' observations and reports of local pressures. The western region's use of needs assessments to provide critical resources, such as information and funds for consultants, is an example of a TQI response to local competitive pressures. Third, the ethical requirements arising from customers', clients', or patients' value systems can be very well understood by applying TQI principles at the regional level or systemwide: visible, ongoing commitment to improvement enhances both patients' and employees' perception that their values and needs are respected. Fourth, TQI implementations, with systemwide or regional support, have overcome the threateningly low JCAHO scores of the mid-1980s. Finally, we observed the snowballing effect of peer pressure on the executives of the region's facilities as adoption of TQI principles spread.

We recognize that there are likely many sources of success in an effort as complex as implementing TQI across a large geographical region and that the region's influence is only one of those sources. For example, many innovations and creative ways of obtaining resources at region facilities may not even have come to regional management's attention. We observe, however, that the region played a strategic role, providing continuous real and symbolic resources during an increasingly challenging time for VA facilities, their leaders, and employees. In applying the region's experience to future large-scale change efforts, it might be useful to consider the model that emerged as we sought to chart and evaluate the implementation of TQI in the West (see Figure 14.1).

Ultimately, TQI implementation in the western region represented the development of an enhanced information and resource distribution system, in which resources and strategic information are pushed to the lowest levels of the organization and knowledge of outcomes flows back up through the organization. The data we have presented here suggest that long-term, sustained commitment may pay off if resource and information flows are kept alive. We know that executives' satisfaction increases with increases in even

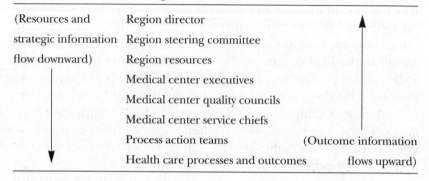

Figure 14.1. A Hierarchical Model of
Western Region Influence and Feedback.

(Resources and	Region director	
strategic information	Region steering committee	
flow downward)	Region resources	
	Medical center executives	
	Medical center quality councils	
	Medical center service chiefs	
	Process action teams	(Outcome information
	Health care processes and outcomes	flows upward)

small amounts of resources and strategic information. And we learned that trained process action teams that were empowered by the opportunity to change strategically important processes were successful. The continuing challenge for the region, for the rest of the VHA health care system, and the nation's health care system as a whole is to keep the feedback process running. That may be the most important long-term benefit of investing in TQI.

References

Berwick, D. M., Godfrey, A. B., & Roessner, J. (1990). *Curing health care: New strategies for quality improvement.* San Francisco: Jossey-Bass.

Imai, M. (1986). *Kaizen: The key to Japan's competitive success.* New York: McGraw-Hill.

Lammers, J. C., Cretin, S., Gilman, S., & Calingo, E. (forthcoming). Findings from a multi-team and multi-hospital study of total quality management: The relationship of leadership and medical staff commitment." *Medical Care.*

Lammers, J. C., & Gilman, S. (1993, December). Quality improvement in VA hospitals: A report on the western region project action teams [Special issue]. *Quality Management in Health Care,* pp. 10–11.

Lammers, J. C., & Gilman, S. (1994a). *Predicting net quality improvement in western region quality improvement teams: Results of a multiple regression analysis.* (Western Region Special Studies Group Technical Report). Washington, DC: Veterans Health Administration.

Lammers, J. C., & Gilman, S. (1994b). *Western region quality improvement and participation in central office implementation phases: A test.* (Western

Region Special Studies Group Technical Report). Washington, DC: Veterans Health Administration.

Lammers, J. C., & Gilman, S. (1995, August). *The quality transformation in VA hospitals.* Proposal submitted to the National Science Foundation, Washington, DC.

Lammers, J. C., Gilman, S., & Calingo, E. (1993). *Quality improvement efforts in western region VA hospitals: Results of a preliminary survey.* (Western Region Special Studies Group Technical Report). Washington, DC: Veterans Health Administration.

Lammers, J. C., Yudelson, J., & Gilman, S. (1995, May 31). *What makes total quality management work? The effect of member homogeneity, training, and team age on perceived quality improvement in hospitals teams.* Paper prepared for the meeting of the International Communication Association, Albuquerque, NM.

Marszalek-Gaucher, E., & Coffey, R. J. (1990). *Transforming healthcare organizations: How to achieve and sustain organizational excellence.* San Francisco: Jossey-Bass.

Tyler, R. (1988, November 14–18). *Quality assurance in the ambulatory care setting.* Paper presented at the annual meeting of the National Institute of Health Care Management, Ft. Lauderdale, FL.

Walton, M. (1986). *The Deming management method.* New York: Putnam.

Chapter Fifteen

The System's Perspective

Linda C. Exner

The thirty-eight medical facilities selected to participate in Phase I and Phase II of the Department of Veterans Affairs' national total quality improvement (TQI) implementation have been the source of a tremendous variety and number of case studies for learning. The foregoing chapters have described how the Veterans Health Administration (VHA) rolled out its TQI process at these medical facilities. In doing so, they illuminated many of the problems and issues that surfaced as individual facilities began to put the principles and processes of TQI in place. This chapter steps back from the description of how TQI was implemented in order to examine these issues from a macro, or system, perspective. From the experiences of Phase I and II sites, the chapter culls various themes and patterns that continue to have a major influence on the evolution of TQI in the VA health care system.

Earlier chapters have described various systemwide issues VHA struggled with even before the TQI rollout started: the national consulting contract, union problems, and the relationship between TQI and quality assurance. As VHA began to implement the basic principles of TQI, many issues began to surface, their full significance obscured by their apparent simplicity. The benefit of hindsight allows us to take a wide-angle view that was not available in the early days. This perspective, in turn, can help us appreciate the true significance of many of the governing principles of TQI:

- Leaders must lead
- Build on what has gone before

- Do not create parallel structures
- Back quality through the system
- Improve quality through teams
- Use quality tools
- Train and do
- Communicate, communicate, communicate

Today, many of these principles are recognized as truisms in the TQI lexicon, dating back to the early days of Dr. W. Edwards Deming. Truisms, however, begin as basic principles and are built on hard-earned experience. These principles were articulated in various VHA TQI training materials and reinforced periodically during the course of the massive TQI training effort. VHA's experiences with these TQI principles, however, strongly suggest that knowing a principle and practicing it are two very different things. Although we knew these principles and some practiced them, as a system we were not diligent in their application. The VA health care system continues to grapple with these principles in its drive to achieve an organizational culture of continuous improvement. The lessons begin at the top, with leadership.

Leaders Must Lead

VHA has traditionally required a very mobile top management team and adaptable field facilities. Top and middle managers are moved about frequently in order to build their knowledge base and experience with the system, as well as to reward, recognize, and take advantage of changing levels of management expertise. During 1992 and 1993, many sites that were involved in the Phase I or II TQI implementation replaced either a director, an associate director, or a chief of staff. Some of the replacements were due to retirements, and others were due to "natural" shifts that occurred secondary to these and other vacancies. Had our TQI culture been in place longer and more widely assimilated into the daily workings of the organization, we might have developed some systemic immunities to these corporate rotations and to what Deming refers to as the "fourth deadly disease . . . mobility of top management" (Walton, 1986, p. 92). As it was, we found ourselves continually fighting organizational barriers and resistance based on the institutional memory of the last "flavor of the month" and the hope that the new leadership would adopt the attitude that "this too shall pass." Additionally, assimilation of the new leaders presented difficulties for sites implementing in Phase I and early Phase II because leadership training and development on TQI philosophy, methodologies, and expectations was not a structured component of the initial implementation model. This lack of uniform and consistent preparation complicated the difficulties experienced by some sites in trying to build momentum.

In retrospect, especially given how highly dependent implementation was on the senior leadership, it seems obvious that much thought and attention should have been given to purposeful, structured preparation of these leaders and other change agents. In the Phase I sites, however, management of implementation roles was essentially dependent on the individuals (internal and external) involved rather than on a structured methodology. For the most part, senior executives and middle managers were not purposefully prepared for the questions, recommendations, and enthusiasm of these participants, or even for the speed with which the implementation process unfolded. They were also ill-prepared as a group to guide the transformation in organizational culture and dynamics that occurred as the change was taking place.

To compound these problems, what attempts *were* made to plan and to prepare organization leaders in an orderly, systematic fashion were sometimes sabotaged by the bureaucracy. For example, plans for an introductory, "kickoff" session for Phase I site leaders and change agents never materialized because of union contract difficulties and repeated delays in the start-up date. By the time the contracts were settled, it was past time to do any advance work, and each site was on its own. The silver lining was that the unused Phase I kickoff funds supported the inclusion of Phase I site leaders in the Phase II kickoff meeting, which did occur preceding the organized start-up of Phase II. Thus Phase I site leaders were able to share with Phase II leaders various pitfalls they had learned from experience, and the Phase II sites certainly benefited from this exchange.

Although there is a natural tendency to remember the pain of failure more than the satisfaction of success, we actually learn as much from success as we do from failure. One of our greatest successes in terms of influencing the needs and methods of leadership development was our early experience with the service quality deployment (SQD) model, which described a step-by-step method for deploying TQI at the service level. In addition, SQD was developed by consultants as a training module targeted at service-level steering committees. The training materials evolved from a mental model used at the Hines VA hospital (the forerunner to the national effort) based on consultant and master trainer feedback from the field. The SQD model was eventually recognized as a microversion of the organizational implementation model used implicitly in consultant interventions with senior staff and facility-level steering committees. Once we discovered what was already in hand, the consultants rapidly converted it into a written *TQI Implementation Guide*. This document was, and continues to be, an invaluable reference for leadership development. Other expressions of this model were developed by the master trainers in collaboration with field staff. The resulting "TQI Implementation Flowchart," "TQI Implementation Advisor," and "TQI Implementation Checklist" have since proven equally valuable and versatile.

One of the primary goals of TQI is to improve quality through a reduction in waste and process variation. Prior to the development of an articulated implementation model and a structured leadership-development program, there was tremendous lack of clarity and much misunderstanding, frustration, and undesirable variation in the systemwide implementation. Collective efforts across the system have resulted in improvements in each of these areas and have provided a common framework that enhances consistency yet allows and encourages local modifications based on each facility's unique culture and circumstances.

Build on What Has Gone Before

Of all the governing principles of TQI noted above, this was the least followed in the Phase I sites. Phase I started at the leading edge of the explosion of total quality applications to the health care industry. Berwick, Godfrey, and Roessner's *Curing Health Care* (1990), the report of the National Demonstration Project's experimental integration of TQI into health care settings, had just been published, as had Marszalek-Gaucher and Coffey's *Transforming*

Healthcare Organizations (1990), an account of the University of Michigan's successful implementation of a total quality framework in its hospital. In general, however, there was very little in the health care literature that demonstrated why and how hospitals should import the successes industrial settings had achieved through adopting total quality methods and mind-sets. By the end of Phase II (the summer and fall of 1993), the literature on TQI had increased profusely, and awareness increased along with it. In addition, when VHA's contract with the American Productivity and Quality Center (APQC) was drafted in 1991, the vast majority of the consultants assigned to the VHA project, although impeccably credentialed in industrial applications of TQI, had minimal, if any, experience implementing it in health care settings. VHA implementation teams, including the master trainers, and hospital leaders were equally inexperienced. Therefore, many of the Phase I sites returned to a relatively "zero" position on the TQI path, without having truly benefited from "quality" and/or "customer-focused" efforts already in place. Of those sites that saw the beginning of TQI in VHA from a different perspective, two best exemplify the range of lessons learned from the principle that TQI changes take time.

The director of the Albany VA medical center, Fred Malphurs, had been preparing the rest of the facility's senior leadership for TQI implementation long before it became a national initiative. Using a low-key but persistent approach, he had been gradually increasing their knowledge and awareness of TQI, by sharing books, journal articles, and his own philosophies. Their chief of staff, Lawrence Flesh, M.D., was a nationally recognized leader in management development for physicians and was a strong proponent of TQI concepts and methods. As students of quality, the Albany staff knew of and understood that the Joint Commission on Accreditation of Healthcare Organizations' (JCAHO) agenda for change was moving toward a continuous quality improvement (CQI) model. Albany's CQI coordinator, Mary Ellen Piché, was already, in 1991, positioning the medical center's quality management activities for these changes. Designating her as the center's executive assistant for TQI sent a very direct message that these quality initiatives would not only not compete with one another, they would be merged from the outset. Even more direct was the

Albany leadership's insistence that TQI be called CQI and that all references and training materials be adapted accordingly. Looking back on those dynamics, it really was an ideal situation for the external consulting "team"—the consultant, physician advisor, and master trainer. The hospital (their customer) knew where it was headed; its leaders were committed to that direction and could negotiate what they wanted to do. They were also open and eager to learn and saw themselves as active partners in the process. They were assertive about adapting the implementation model to their local needs and not only "building on what had gone before" but also building toward their future vision of an integrated quality effort. Although they had not really conceptualized themselves as a team or a partnership, those early days in which they constructed the "Albany Model" forged that kind of relationship. The identification of a common purpose, the discovery of each individual's unique abilities to contribute to that purpose, and the excitement and energy generated by these were the essential elements from which the team was built. The ability to truly "meet the customers where they were" provided numerous process examples that were adapted and adopted systemwide. Although Albany probably had the internal strength to succeed on its own, the synergy that resulted from the expansion of its capabilities through external TQI supports is seen as a significant factor in the speed of their success. Albany was recognized for its outstanding accomplishments when it was awarded the Robert W. Carey Quality Award in 1993. This award is the Department of Veterans Affairs equivalent of the President's Award for Quality; it is modeled after the Malcolm Baldrige Quality Award and is the most prestigious award for quality in VA.

The Indianapolis VA hospital, also a Phase I site, won the Robert W. Carey Quality Award, health care category, in 1994. Although the results at Albany and Indianapolis were similar and both won a prestigious quality award, the Indianapolis story provides a different perspective (as well as a strong reinforcement of the "build on what has gone before" principle).

At Indianapolis, the vision and commitment of the senior leadership was also evident long before the national initiative began. In 1988, they began a pilot TQI program, working with a different consulting firm from the one chosen for VHA's national rollout. By April of 1991, six months before the official Phase I start-up, the

Indianapolis facility had three cross-functional process action teams going, and it was preparing to launch nine more (Honen, 1991). They had trained extensive numbers of staff using their consulting firm's materials, which used a different performance improvement model and vernacular than the materials APQC was developing for VHA. Following a series of unsuccessful attempts to forge a partnership with the national consulting team that would build on these efforts, Indianapolis decided not to use the consulting support available under the national contract. They continued to participate in the TQI network that was beginning to form across the system as well as in other systemwide activities and events. Their withdrawal from the national consulting program freed up resources to provide consulting support to a different VA hospital. Like Albany, this customer knew what it wanted and was willing to engage in partnership, but (justifiably) not at the risk of having to rebuild any of what it had already accomplished.

Like the other Phase I pilot sites, the Indianapolis and Albany VA hospitals were chosen not because of their deficiencies but because of their high probability of achieving success. Indeed, both of these facilities had already been highly successful. While Albany benefited from its participation in the pilot phase, Indianapolis clearly succeeded independently of the national initiative. The dynamics common to both were a strong and visible commitment to TQI from visionary leaders and an insistence on the integration of any new efforts within their existing quality improvement framework.

The story of these two sites has been somewhat oversimplified to illustrate the principle of building on what has gone before. Their stories represent two different approaches, the dynamics and how-tos of which have been as varied and complex among VHA sites as the sites themselves.

Do Not Create Parallel Structures

A major influence on the structure, functioning, and even the very existence of hospitals and other medical care facilities is exerted by the Joint Commission on Accreditation of Healthcare Organizations (JCAHO). Unfortunately, this influence is too often regarded as punitive and undesirable rather than guiding and exemplary. These views may lead to managers' missing or, at best, underestimating important shifts in philosophies and quality management trends. One such shift could have been used by VHA as a cornerstone of its TQI vision. In 1986, JCAHO began publicizing its "agenda for change," a proposed revision of its accreditation standards, which ostensibly grew out of many of the socioeconomic changes that occurred in health care earlier in the decade. The focus of the commission's new evaluation methodology was to be continuous improvement of clinical and organizational performance. It was to be based on an array of clinical and organizational performance indicators to be developed and tested over the next several years. The study of organizational indicators was expected to lead to improved accreditation standards; standards "that are demonstrably important to the provision of quality patient care" (Lehmann, 1987) and "provide a foundation for continual improvement" (Joint Commission on Accreditation of Healthcare Organizations, 1990). By 1990, the many operational and corporate changes that were sweeping the business world, including numerous non–health care service industries, could have provided a backdrop for VHA's interpretation of the JCAHO accreditation changes, thereby acting as a springboard for TQI. Perhaps the language was too new. For whatever reasons, no organizational position on this was built into VHA's initial TQI model.

Without a clear direction from the national level, the fundamental problem of failing to "build on what has gone before" affected the structures and systems that evolved naturally from the parallel TQI/CQI track we found ourselves on in many facilities. Several important and ongoing facility functions, including quality management, strategic planning, and customer satisfaction initiatives were not, except in rare instances, initially integrated with the TQI efforts in Phase I and early Phase II. If the potential reasons for this were arranged on an Ishikawa diagram, major categories might include the following:

1. *The model.* The consultants' general inexperience with health care's quality heritage and the richness and complexity of "Q" in this context, and the subsequent considerations this should have been given in the implementation model.

2. *Politics.* Hardened silos at all levels of the bureaucracy, from local facilities to headquarters and including the major (and sometimes adversarial) divisions between administrative and clinical, line and staff, and organized labor and management.

3. *Positioning.* From the onset of Phase I through the early to mid stages of Phase II, the locus of control (funding, programmatic oversight, decision making, and resource allocation) for TQI was in the Office of Resource Management at VHA headquarters. While this served the very beneficial function of identifying this as "not just another quality assurance program," visible (from the field) links to the Office of Quality Management were very weak, at best. Local facilities were encouraged to position their TQI effort under their own director rather than under the chief of staff (to whom about 50 percent of the quality management programs in the system reported). While this was intended to "elevate" the status of TQI, to highlight leadership's role, and to reinforce its universality, it often unintentionally reinforced negative perceptions of quality management and left room for facilities to choose to keep these initiatives separate.

4. *Perceptions.* TQI and CQI/quality management (QM) were intentionally separated in many facilities in order to avoid any negative associations carried over from the traditional quality management focus on uncovering "bad apples" and correcting poor quality through interventions geared at improving individual (rather than process) performance.

5. *The players.* Most of the key players in the implementation did not start out in a "bicultural," TQI/QM mode. Many did not even speak the other's language, much less think in an integrated fashion. In most cases, the external consultants took a neutral position (either due to their lack of technical expertise or their need to remain process-focused in order to achieve facility buy-in); in a few instances, the external consultant(s) actually advocated the parallel track.

These and many other variables contributed to VHA's finding itself well into Phase II before changes of enough significance had occurred in the dynamics listed previously to produce a shift in organizational philosophy to an integrated model. Fortunately, there was a significant, though minority, core of individuals who recognized this need from the outset and were working within their own spheres of influence (field facilities, regional medical education centers, continuing education centers, consulting firms, and headquarters) to develop whatever was necessary to bridge the gaps and eliminate any avoidable duplication. Among these, it was the quality managers and executive assistants for TQI with an integrated vision who struggled the most with these issues and who developed the innovative structures and strategies that are now mutating throughout the system as we move toward a fully integrated effort. Another major catalyst in the integration occurred when the responsibility for TQI was shifted away from resource management and into the Office of Quality Management. This formalized, strengthened, and expanded the many collaborative efforts that were already under way between staff that had been artificially divided by their reporting relationship within the organization. In addition, this alliance began to rid the system of some of its redundancy in "quality" initiatives, thus freeing up resources and energy for the enormous and ever-increasing needs of the system as a whole.

Back Quality Through the System

The fundamental premise behind this principle is that quality *must* be defined by customer expectations, needs, and requirements. This is consistent with Stephen Covey's second principle of effectiveness, which urges managers to "begin with the end in mind" (Covey, 1989, p. 95). In TQI, identification of customer requirements is considered to be the essential first step in any process improvement, redesign, or reengineering. Differences between what the customer needs and expects and what the organization actually delivers are defined as "performance gaps" or "opportunities for improvement." This kind of thinking was very new and very alien to VHA's culture in 1991. We learned much about organizational culture, particularly resistance to change and organizational reinforcement of the prevailing culture, when we attempted to alter the organizational definition of quality.

Although a customer focus was very much the center of industrial total quality management (TQM) and was reinforced under Secretary Derwinski's administration through the establishment of the Robert W. Carey Quality Award and the TQI initiative, VHA had some major barriers to overcome. The first hurdle was an immediate and vociferous objection to the term *customer* and all that it implied. These objections were mostly heard from direct care providers, particularly physicians. We were not in a sales business, they said; our patients didn't "pay" for their care like they would pay for a car, for example; even third-party reimbursements were not an integral part of the VHA system. But most of all, the term *customer* was demeaning to the patient-provider relationship. Although the concepts, not the semantics, were the critical issues, the general uproar over terminology raged for some time. Perhaps this was partially symptomatic of a deep vein of resistance to TQI concepts and the fundamental role shifts that would be one consequence of accepting the model. Some may have perceived this shift in semantics as a beginning use of business practices, which would undermine the autonomy of clinical decision makers. These role shifts would not only affect relationships with the external customers and suppliers, they would fundamentally reorder the way in which employees related to one another.

VA hospitals, like most other health care organizations, had a traditional organizational structure with a major division between "professional" (clinical) and administrative and other support services. In addition to this overt structure, the culture of health care facilities is also based on a complex caste system that governs the balance of power in the organization. Identification of an individual employee's place within that system is readily made through the visual label of their work attire; from short to long white coats and all other colors of uniforms to the variations in the formality of the nonuniformed. In the customer-supplier model, traditional hierarchy and power relationships are meaningless. The customer is king or queen. To complicate matters, in health care, as with other service industries, these relationships are nonlinear and changing, not only with specific processes but also within processes. In fact, it is not unusual for one to be both a customer as well as a supplier in the same process. For example, the patient who receives a blood transfusion (the "customer") very often is the one who donated the blood (the "supplier"). The doctor who orders the blood (a "copartner" of the primary customer) also "supplies" all the relevant details of the conditions under which the blood should be given (process requirements). These customer-supplier dynamics and the perceived risks and benefits of the new relationships were revealed as significant factors in the transfer and acceptance of the new technology.

There were (and are) many people in VHA, as in any health care setting, whose past life experience has taught them that revealing "bad" outcomes leads to "punishment" (and, in some cases, litigation), not to "opportunities for improvement." This has been reinforced by the traditional quality assurance (QA) and QM focus on individual versus process or system performance and the search for "bad apples." We learned in the early phases that it does take time, patience, and, most of all, continual reinforcement through consistent and congruent messages from the leadership and other significant individuals to overwrite a learned avoidance to "negative" feedback. Deming cites "driving out fear" as one of his essential "14 points" (Walton, 1986, p. 35). This is much harder to accomplish in a highly regulated, highly visible, high-stakes industry where a certain amount of fear is considered essential to self-preservation. However, open feedback systems and honest data are even more essential.

Our grasp of these issues and the system's response to them has become more and more congruent with the principle of "backing quality through the system" over the course of time. A major reinforcement of this principle has been the vision and examples set by the Clinton administration's secretary for the Department of Veterans Affairs, Jesse Brown. As part of an administration that pledged to bring customer-focused reform to the federal government, Mr. Brown quickly established and communicated a vision that put the focus of the department's efforts on the veteran and his or her family. In addition, he has kept the message of "putting veterans first" in front of the workforce in a variety of ways.

What was, in 1991, a foreign concept that was vigorously opposed by staff has now become accepted, if not normative. The lessons learned from this include a better understanding of the dynamics and issues surrounding cultural change and the importance of both attending to concerns as well as communicating expectations and developing reward and reinforcement systems that are congruent with the desired change.

Improve Quality Through Teams

We learned the value of this principle over and over in our early transition into a TQI framework. Although we initially thought of process action teams as the primary illustration of this principle, as our knowledge and understanding of implementation demands grew, so did our reliance on teams that could provide a much broader spectrum of contributions to the implementation effort. The following examples of structures that were not initially conceptualized as "teams" but, in fact, needed to function in that manner best illustrate the team lessons learned in Phases I and II.

In the "Leaders Must Lead" section above, we spoke of the center- and service-level oversight structures initially referred to as quality steering committees. As our experience grew, it became apparent that the term *quality leadership team* (QLT) was far more descriptive of both the desired role of these structures and of how the groups themselves would best function. Those functioning under the name *steering committee* were thought to be more likely to fall into a traditional management-versus-leadership paradigm and be more prone to acting hierarchically rather than in an egalitarian, team fashion. Calling these groups leadership teams reflected our growing awareness of the real value of teams versus other kinds of groups.

Another example of our recognition and internalization of this value occurred with the "core four," the group composed of the APQC consultant, the physician advisor, the RMEC master trainer (the three external consultants), and the facility-based executive assistant for TQI (an internal consultant). As noted earlier, this group was billed as the implementation team. However, as with the facility leadership groups, no formal structure existed to develop these individuals as a team. Consequently, in most of the Phase I sites they *did not* function as a team. Not only were their roles not clearly defined in Phase I but most, if not all, of the external players were in various stages of readiness with respect to the content and technical expertise required to fulfill the contract's obligations. Those who reached out informally to their other "team" members rapidly reinforced what the teams under their direction and guidance were discovering; that while each individual may not have the entire package required for success, their collective knowledge and experience was extremely powerful. By the time of the Phase II kickoff, the successful team roles that had emerged and were evolving in the Phase I pilot sites were legitimized and presented to Phase II leaders. This not only communicated the realistic expectations of the external consultants to the Phase II sites but also reinforced to those directly involved what had been learned through the successes and failures of the Phase I sites.

Another value of team dynamics in TQI organizations is self-direction. The master trainer group is a good example of how self-direction can naturally emerge through teamwork and participative management. The master trainer group has been coordinated since its inception by Lynn Ward, the program director at the St. Louis continuing education center (CEC). Through her leadership, the master trainers have been encouraged to evolve into a quasi-self-directed work team around a variety of tasks. As individuals as well as members of inter-RMEC and cross-functional teams, master trainers have attended to the multiple tasks and duties associated with the education and training demands of the national effort. In addition, they have recognized and acted on opportunities to collaborate, share lessons learned, and continuously improve materials and approaches to training. They have also supported one another through the training and development stages of Phases I and II, and they continue to provide peer review and assistance for the complex challenges we are experiencing in the later phases. Formal training in intentional interventions to produce team self-direction is now an option in the "advanced toolbox."

Use Quality Tools

If "build on what has gone before" was the least applied principle of TQI, then the principle of "use quality tools" was perhaps the least understood. But it is also an area in which we have made substantial progress. In the TQI training materials, this principle primarily refers to the "seven basic tools" for the graphical depiction and analysis of quantitative data. The principle's full power is realized, however, through the scope and depth of the array of quantitative and qualitative tools used in the implementation. These are learned somewhat inductively through their application to specific tasks. The tools include matrices, decision grids, and other structured guides that assist in generating and organizing ideas, opinions, and other qualitative data needed to make choices and optimize decision making. Even the "ordinary" and "common sense" tools of agendas and minutes are considered to be essential components of a complete TQI toolbox. However, some of the most ordinary tools are the most difficult to use. The flowchart is a good example.

VHA TQI teams are taught a process for improvement that includes three phases: understand, analyze, and improve. Following the identification of customer requirements, the mandatory second step to achieve understanding is to flowchart the process, adding shape and substance through an ancillary technique referred to as process definition. This is a methodology for identifying the customer-supplier relationships of the various steps within the process. As previously discussed, lack of a clearly defined structure and process for the TQI implementation hindered our initial activities in the pilot sites and contributed to much avoidable confusion and variation. Once a process was identified, the process steps could be ordered, described, and flowcharted. The resulting "implementation flowchart" became the simplified road map that communicated the steps to be followed and served to reduce unwanted variation. In addition, the identification of the major process steps aided in identifying customer groups within this process, subsequently facilitating opportunities to continuously improve the model (see "Back Quality Through the System," above). In addition to numerous other system improvements realized through the use of basic tools, system improvements have also been achieved using more advanced tools, such as quality function deployment (QFD) and benchmarking.

QFD, the use of teams of individuals who will be affected by the process (including customers and suppliers), is a highly profitable method of building quality into a new or reengineered process. Although the wisdom and utility of this proactive technique was recognized fairly early, we were well into Phase II before we began to incorporate it in any substantive way. Based on the lessons learned from the rework that had to be done when customer input was not built into the design of a product or service delivery process, we began to use QFD methods for emerging product and service lines in the national TQI inventory. Examples of this included the executive assistant college and new executive assistant orientation programs, additional courses such as "Coaching and Mentoring" and "Internal Consulting Skills," and initiatives to build the system infrastructure for networking and benchmarking. In each of these, teams composed of field staff (customers), APQC and/or RMEC staff (suppliers), and those who would directly participate in the process were formed to design and pilot the products and services.

Train and Do

The rollout of TQI in VHA was designed to benefit from the timely, positive outcomes resulting from the principle "train and do." Training is most useful if it is related to an individual's needs and if it is "just-in-time," that is, immediately applicable to an individual's life. Implementing TQI in an organization presents multiple and ongoing opportunities for relevant, applicable training. Of the four core TQI courses offered in VHA, only "TQI Awareness" did not immediately precede or involve actual hands-on activity. "Awareness" was targeted at all employees and was designed to be offered as a general, introductory course. It was typically structured in short (one- to two-hour) sessions that included not only basic TQI concepts but also a briefing on local TQI implementation activities and time lines. The other three core courses, however, were taught interactively, and many of the concepts and theories presented were illustrated through the completion of real-world tasks and activities integrated into the training agenda. The goal was to give those being trained, the process improvement and senior-level leadership teams and their team leaders and facilitators, a head start with their assignments.

Master trainer training also followed the "train and do" prescription. Master trainers were selected and their training and "apprenticeship" started only when Phase I sites were ready to implement TQI. This learning experience included elements of both classroom and on-the-job training and development. By the end of Phase I, twenty master trainers had been hired, and most were at least partway through the required training program. At each Phase II site, the master trainers also followed the "train and do" directive, with their goal being to leave each site on its own with a full complement of certified trainers who could carry on with local training and certification as needed. Training is an essential part of implementing any new program or process in an organization, and making it as meaningful as possible is the best way to be effective.

Communicate, Communicate, Communicate

Many examples of the principle "communicate, communicate, communicate" could be observed in Phases I and II. Because the VHA system spans the entire nation, its need for both intra- and interagency communication is not surprising. The fact that effective communication is critical to a TQI effort was well known, and VHA endeavored to practice it from the outset. Many individual sites used relatively common local communication mechanisms such as newsletters, bulletin boards, team storyboard displays, and all-staff meetings; however, the focus of this section is on systemwide efforts that made a difference in the growth and development of the many types of individuals involved in the TQI implementation. Methodologies ranged from the traditional to the more contemporary and include the writing of this book so that VHA's story could be told to an even wider audience.

As noted, the activity center of the TQI-related communication effort was in the educational support office at the St. Louis CEC. In addition to the time they spent together for training and work sessions, master trainers "met" on a monthly basis via telephone conference calls to share ideas and news and to begin planning for new activities. The executive assistants for TQI also met quarterly via conference call; however, their calls were more planned and were structured to meet continuing education needs that had already been expressed. The regular conference calls continue to this day for these groups. E-mail was another major communication tool that is still used extensively. A somewhat restricted E-mail group was established for master trainers, executive assistants, and other individuals involved in implementing TQI at the national level. Most VHA employees are very familiar with E-mail and are quite comfortable with signing in and engaging in a free exchange of ideas. This mail group became a rich source of information as new people were introduced and welcomed, questions or concerns were posted and answered, and new ideas were put forth for consideration. Many individuals grew to know others in the system via E-mail long before they ever knew what they looked like or how they sounded. The mail groups continue to be highly active and very successful and have only grown in number.

The CEC also became a clearinghouse for paper-based information; many exchanges of such information are initiated by E-mail requests for information that receive a long series of "me, too" requests. The CEC eventually became a collection and distribution center for articles, newsletters, reports, white papers, plans, and progress notes, which were sent across the nation on a regular basis. One other method of communication that was practiced as often as possible involved sharing successes and lessons learned from the individual sites. Whenever a national or regional conference related to TQI was planned, an opportunity was offered for "show-and-tell" sessions to relate individual stories, and space was made available for displays that could be viewed throughout the conference. Because of the ongoing success of all of these communications methods, plans were under way near the end of Phase II to develop more formal networking and benchmarking protocols so the entire system could benefit from individual and shared lessons learned.

Even though the need for interagency communication was not new to VHA and the tools and technology to make good communication a reality were readily available, the underlying lesson related to this principle may be that the heart and soul of good communication is people. If people who need information or who have information to share aren't willing to become involved with and actively participate in a communication network, having the network in place won't matter.

Conclusion

As we look back on Phases I and II through the filter of experience and the lens of the current environment, it is clear that, while all the lessons learned were important, the most significant lesson has been in the art and science of thinking and acting as a system. Peter Senge describes this as the "fifth discipline" of a "learning organization" (Senge, 1990, p. 12). Our lessons learned represent many of the component elements of the five disciplines described by Senge. The TQI implementation effort has required a systematic, systemic mind-set and approach to transcend the many parochial boundaries within VHA. These efforts will continue to prepare the culture and provide many of the major tools for the next major step in VHA's transformation into a customer-driven, significant player in the competitive health care market of the twenty-first century. The ability to continue to learn and grow as a system within this larger context will be essential to not just VHA's but to any health care organization's success.

References

Berwick, D. M., Godfrey, A. B., & Roessner, J. (1990). *Curing health care: New strategies for quality improvement.* San Francisco: Jossey-Bass.

Covey, S. R. (1989). *The seven habits of highly effective people.* New York: Simon & Schuster.

Honen, D. (1991, April). Richard L. Roudebush VAMC, Indianapolis, Indiana: Health care with a new look. *VA Practitioner,* pp. 35–48.

Joint Commission on Accreditation of Healthcare Organizations. (1990). The Joint Commission's agenda for change: Stimulating continual improvement in the quality of care. Chicago: Author.

Lehmann, R. D. (1987, April). Joint Commission sets agenda for change. *Quality Review Bulletin,* pp. 148–150.

Marszalek-Gaucher, E., & Coffey, R. J. (1990). *Transforming healthcare organizations: How to achieve and sustain organizational excellence.* San Francisco: Jossey-Bass.

Senge, P. M. (1990). *The fifth discipline: The art and practice of the learning organization.* New York: Doubleday.

Walton, M. (1986). *The Deming management method.* New York: Putnam.

Chapter Sixteen

Setting the Stage for the Future

Lynn D. Ward

When plans for major change efforts are developed, the vision of "what should be" inevitably butts up against reality, and revisions must be made. Shortly after the Phase II rollout began in June 1992, VHA's TQI coordinating committee began to plan the Phase III rollout, which was to involve forty-eight sites yet to be selected. In the context of that planning activity, it became evident that the original plan for the implementation of TQI in VHA needed to be adapted to fit the needs of the system and to support the reality that had developed from the first two phases. Four major issues surfaced that required new approaches:

- A need to decentralize the TQI effort
- A need to speed up the rollout in order to respond to various efforts initiated by sites not included in Phases I and II
- The reassignment of responsibility for the TQI program from the Office of Resource Management to the Office of Quality Management
- A recognition that a major transfer to in-house capability was not taking place as planned

In addition, as hospitals and staff became more experienced in pursuing TQI, we identified content areas that needed to be explored, presented, and supported that were beyond our original plans.

The impact of the unfair labor practice action filed by the American Federation of Government Employees (AFGE) union was discussed in an earlier chapter. The TQI coordinating committee did not want to lose the momentum that had been gained at individual facilities while waiting for this issue to resolve. We looked at methodologies that would make sure the process was decentralized, with much more local determination and no appreciable centralized direction. If all of the support already in place were cut off, the medical centers would have to assume much more of the cost, do without essential support elements, or some combination of these two choices. Several steps were taken to ensure both that TQI was a locally determined management philosophy and that needed support would still be available to keep the implementation on track.

A major change in organizational responsibility was necessary because of the union's charges. If TQI were truly to be "decentralized," the primary program owner could no longer be the Office of Resource Management. The decision was made to transfer the responsibilities to the TQI Coordinating Committee, with the operational aspects of the rollout to be housed at the St. Louis continuing education center (CEC). The committee was reconfigured to include more field than headquarters representatives and to exclude outside consultants; its major responsibility was to set directions for the development of VHA support and TQI infrastructure, but it had no line authority over the medical centers.

We perceived that the centralized consulting contract would be a major stumbling block if we were to move to a decentralized program. With some concern about the outcomes, the TQI committee decided that the money available for the contract would be given to the medical centers; they would decide what consultants they would work with and would write their own contracts. The money could have been divided equally between all of the sites; however, based on our experiences to that point, we assumed not all hospitals were equal in their commitment to TQI. We wanted to ensure that the money went to facilities that wanted to implement TQI and had a plan to do so; therefore, we wanted to build in some variation in dollars awarded to each site based on measurable criteria.

Each site not designated as a Phase I or II site was asked if it wanted to take part in Phase III; if so, they were to complete a checklist of their TQI efforts and intentions, forward a statement of commitment written by the medical center director, address their willingness to collaborate with other sites in training events, and define how they would spend the money they would receive. A review panel of ten people from the system (from the field and from the central office) met, set the specific evaluation criteria, reviewed the proposals, and rated the sites, dividing the available money at three different levels of funding. As soon as the medical centers could provide us with specifics (that is, tell us what they would purchase with the money and from whom), the money was transferred to them.

The centralized consulting contract stipulated that the consulting group was responsible for ensuring that TQI activities were accomplished. Specific areas in the work agreement that would now need to be addressed differently included training and development of VA facility leaders; development of networking capabilities; identification of benchmark organizations and processes, both within and outside VHA; and the planning of systemwide workshops or national meetings.

Developing Infrastructure Within the New Decentralized Plan

Since each VA facility would now approach TQI independently, there was an increased need for support structures that would enable them to implement TQI; it was a challenge for the central office to develop support for this task that would be helpful but not directive.

John Fears recognized that activities that had been the responsibility of the program office still needed to be accomplished, but without central office control or ownership. He requested that the regional medical education center (RMEC) council establish committees to look at needs that spanned the individual facilities. The following committees would report to the TQI Coordinating Committee:

- *Networking and benchmarking committee.* This committee would be charged with supporting TQI networking and benchmarking within VHA by assessing the effectiveness of existing activities, testing various ways to perform these functions, and making recommendations on policy and practices to the VHA central office.
- *Newsletter and other publications committee.* Originally seen as two committees, this single entity would publish a quarterly newsletter for systemwide distribution and would capture information recognizing excellence in process action teams for publication.
- *Evaluation and measurement committee.* This committee would be responsible for designing and implementing various evaluation and measurement schemes for use by VA facilities in evaluating the effects of their TQI processes.

In early 1993, the TQI program office moved from the Office of Resource Management to the Office of Quality Management. VHA leaders had concluded that the failure to tie TQI and QM together at the central office allowed—indeed, exacerbated—the inefficient and frequently divisive separation of "quality" activities at the individual medical centers. The move to the Office of Quality Management underscored the recognition that the activities of traditional quality assurance or quality management (QM) and TQI were inextricably related and should be integrated at the medical centers. The staffing and alignment of the positions were left to the medical centers, but the need to ensure that TQI and QM proceeded in concert at all levels was now officially stated, in many ways.

Numerous activities and collaborative efforts were initiated to support the integration of TQI and QM activities and practices. Training material was reviewed and rewritten. Hospital QM coordinators were involved in TQI activities, and executive assistants for TQI (EAs) were involved in QM activities and meetings. Funding was provided for eight sites to develop site models for TQI/QM integration.

As noted earlier, the hospitals to be included in Phase III and Phase IV were not selected from the original requests for proposals. Thus we needed to identify the Phase III sites before we could proceed. But as we began to move in that direction, we found that more and more hospitals had begun TQI on their own, without waiting to become an official site. There were diverse reasons for this "self-starting" of TQI. In some cases, the leaders were convinced of the value of applying TQI concepts to help their organization deal with the changing health care environment. Business leaders like Ritz-Carlton and Chrysler were demonstrating the value of basic TQI concepts in a competitive environment. Health care leaders were applying TQI principles successfully and going public to share the new "religion." The surge in TQI implementation nationwide was evidenced by the book *Curing Health Care* (Berwick, Godfrey, & Roessner, 1990), which described the experiences of the National Demonstration Project; by the American College of Healthcare Executives training courses covering such topics as clinical pathways, reorganization, and TQI support; and by the emergence of new TQI experts across the country. Lay periodicals such as *U.S. News and World Report* and *Business Week* featured stories or entire issues devoted to TQI in health care ("America's Best Hospitals," 1993; "The Quality Imperative," 1991; "Quality: How to Make it Pay," 1994). It was now evident to even the casual observer that the Joint Commission for the Accreditation of Healthcare Organizations (JCAHO) was moving in this direction. While JCAHO emphasized that it would not demand TQI implementation, it was clear that it was going to evaluate VA facilities against such standards as "leaders are trained in continuous improvement"—standards that would require evidence of the integration of continuous improvement outcomes and plans into centers' budgets, of the establishment of cross-functional teams to collect data (measurements) to indicate needed changes, and of efforts to make the necessary corrections. But whatever the stimulus, the medical centers were moving ahead in TQI efforts on their own.

Events beyond our control had changed the environment. Some variation in the original plan was mandatory; the challenge was to foster success within the limitations now present. The TQI Coordinating Committee identified the following two options:

1. *Continue with the initial rollout schedule, and focus on only forty-eight additional sites.* Those sites that were going ahead on their own

would continue as they started, without becoming part of the systemwide TQI effort. In fact, at that point, we were excluding non–Phase I and II sites from attending centralized training or meetings and from using the materials we had developed and printed. This option would continue that exclusionary approach, because of a lack of a common approach. Thus, VA hospitals across the system would pursue various models of implementation, without a common infrastructure or support. There would be little or no transportability of experiences, lessons learned, training, or trainers from one site to another.

2. *Bring the remaining sites (as many as 140) into Phase III, and lengthen the phase to two years.* Each site would receive less money and less human assistance than in Option 1 (that is, the contracting budget had been set a year ago, based on forty-eight sites, and there were only twenty master trainers available to work with the medical centers and provide training). The advantages to this choice would be that we would offer the same assistance to everyone, increasing the likelihood of common approaches, terminology, even internal organization; that we would assist all who wanted our help; that we would not exclude sites; and that the medical centers would have more say in their own implementation process. However, we would need to rewrite our plan to respond to the new shape of the project.

The TQI Coordinating Committee decided that the only feasible choice was to enlarge Phase III to encompass all the sites that wanted to take part. The sites were moving ahead, and if we wanted to be their leader, we had to get out in front and incorporate all of their approaches into a systemwide initiative.

Since the master trainers needed to train trainers in more hospitals (140 rather than 38), we had to devise a way to present training to more than one hospital at a time. We established centralized or cluster training events for twenty-five to thirty participants; the training was held at each RMEC for the hospitals in its catchment area. This allowed three trainers (per RMEC) to conduct the first round of training (the core TQI course) for all of the hospitals in a catchment area simultaneously. The master trainers could then work with each site individually to continue the development of the trainers and to certify selected individuals as local master trainers.

The consultants had conducted leadership conferences for Phase I and Phase II sites. The TQI Coordinating Committee directed the TQI training committee to assume leadership in developing training sessions for the sites choosing to participate in Phase III. The conference was designed for directors, chiefs of staff, EAs, and quality managers from each of the sites; included updated information regarding TQI implementation in VHA; featured nationally recognized experts in TQI and customer service; provided skills training; and presented structured networking activities.

The original implementation plan was based on transferring capability for training and consultation to VHA personnel so that dependence on outside consultants would quickly diminish. The master trainers and many of the EAs were becoming certified as trainers and as trainers of trainers as scheduled. Additional courses were being developed and delivered. The transfer of training appeared to be on track.

However, the consulting capability was not being developed as anticipated. A key to tutoring the EAs for TQI was the plan for them (in Phase II, III, and IV) to learn along with the earlier, Phase I EAs so that they would be prepared to facilitate TQI at their site prior to actual start-up. The point was important because in each phase the EAs received half as much external consulting time as they had in the prior phase. This major shortcoming, combined with the further diminished resources for Phase III (and the old Phase IV) sites, resulted in some EAs having minimal expertise, despite their being expected to serve as internal TQI resources. A second concern was the broad variance in the individuals chosen to fulfill the EA function. The individuals came in various shapes, diverse in background, grade, collateral responsibilities, even roles. We could identify no single approach that would prepare the EAs to assume the consulting roles within the limitations set on us by the budget lines.

The members of the TQI Coordinating Committee faced a conundrum as they grappled with the role of the EA. Discussion was agonized and heated as they faced the inevitable trade-off between better-prepared EAs in the original plan and less-prepared EAs in the speeded-up plan. On the one hand, we could have kept to the original plan and developed it better, but the original plan was becoming more and more moot as individual hospitals embarked on their solitary TQI journeys. This was little solace to the potential Phase IV sites when they were told that they would have to wait almost two more years for any formal support. Thus, the decision to merge Phases III and IV was made with the full realization that there would be some attrition in the ranks of EAs and an increased likelihood of unsuccessful implementation at some sites.

Therefore, when we adapted the original plan, most of our effort was focused on developing the internal consulting capability of the EAs to the maximum extent possible. The first modification was to provide additional training and assistance to them in a concentrated manner. We formed a task force to look at the issue of EA development, to identify the knowledge and skills needed and to find or develop training opportunities for them. The task force began to build a structure for an EA college, a combination of experiences and courses that could be designed to meet the needs of the individual EA. A new course, Internal Consulting, was developed in collaboration with the consultants and made available to the EAs. The networking and benchmarking committee promoted the use of on-site visits, or "mini-residencies," for EAs to learn firsthand from an experienced EA and to directly observe the TQI activities at a site that had been at this business for a period of time. The TQI national training program budgeted money to pay for the travel involved in these networking events.

National forums were also developed and conducted. The EAs and quality managers from all VA facilities across the country came together for three days of information, skill building, and networking opportunities. The participants included faculty as well as students. They presented information about their experiences through various formats and were eager to learn from their colleagues.

We also decided to prepare a cadre of individuals to serve as internal VHA consultants to work with the medical centers as they progressed through their TQI implementation. We wanted individuals who had a good knowledge of TQI concepts and skills, possessed experience in or with the medical centers, and would be available to assist at other sites. We found that the master trainers were beginning to take on some of these responsibilities already and certainly met the criteria listed. Therefore, we designed a method for pairing TQI team leaders at each RMEC with American Productivity and Quality Center (APQC) consultants at sites starting up TQI during the revised Phase III. We offered a special grant to twelve sites: we would match funds the medical centers invested, sufficient to purchase twenty-seven consulting days (generally nine 3-day visits) from APQC. (The amount awarded to these sites was two to five times the money given to other Phase III sites.) Our requirement for the investment was an agreement from the site and the consultant that the master trainer would be included in scheduling and conducting the consultation activities and that the consultant would be tutoring him or her to assume similar consulting responsibilities at other sites. The facility benefited by receiving additional funding for consultants and by having two "outside experts" at the site for each visit, multiplying the benefit to the site.

As stated in the introduction, throughout Phase I and then Phase II, we were learning of related content areas that needed further modification or needed to be developed and made available to facilities in an organized manner. The following list is not inclusive, but it addresses major areas of effort, courses, and/or products:

- *Benchmarking.* Benchmarking would become increasingly important to VHA as it looked ahead to the changes taking place in health care; VHA would be developing services not previously delivered. Business leaders had profited significantly from benchmarking activities. Benchmarking is key to making major changes, to developing new processes (product lines), and to efforts to become "best in the business."
- *Strategic planning.* The first phases of the TQI implementation had included development of strategic plans at each site. Leadership at the facilities and within our coordinating committee recognized that strategic planning needed to be revisited as the facilities moved from looking at improving what they were doing to entering into new delivery and funding models, as well as responding to the expectations of their health care "customers."
- *Customer service.* We recognized the agency's increased emphasis on customer focus and expectations (as underlined by the

secretary's program of "putting veterans first"). TQI is built on identifying customers and designing all activities and processes with that in mind. However, this was a time to reemphasize the importance of listening to the customer and responding to his or her message. We looked for ways to incorporate information from the national patient survey, now being conducted by the National Customer Feedback Center, and from the Federal Quality Institute's "Creating a Customer-Focused Government" training materials.

• *Team database.* The networking and benchmarking committee initiated development of a computerized database containing essential information about process improvement teams established in VA facilities nationwide. The database can be accessed by individuals at any VHA site. All sites were invited to enter information on their teams and to look at information from other sites. VHA and non-VHA groups had identified a need for a user-friendly, timely way to share information about teams already in place, which would diminish the need to start all over each time sites approach common processes needing improvement.

• *Facilitation skills.* Sites identified the need for additional training and skill building for team facilitators. The team training materials would be supplemented, with still greater supplementation for facilitators. The master trainers shared information about development of site-specific support groups for facilitators.

• *Development for mid-level managers.* The original implementation model provided little training specifically for supervisors and service chiefs. Generally they received training only when they served on the quality leadership team, on specific process action teams, or in a service quality deployment capacity. As discussed earlier, this was a major omission—these were the individuals who were leading the majority of the workforce, who were setting the culture in which the anticipated improvements were to take place. Recognizing the need to help managers transition from old ways of supervising and doing business to the skills and approaches needed in a TQI culture, we developed new courses and materials in the areas of coaching, mentoring, and working with self-directed work teams.

• *Additional support materials.* We found in Phase I that leaders at the individual medical centers were looking for something—

a document, a map, some sort of reference—that would describe what was going to happen at their site as they started TQI and continued TQI implementation. The materials used in core TQI courses explained TQI concepts, key components, and skills, but they did not lay out the complete picture or describe what to expect next. We worked with the consultants to develop a notebook composed of modules addressing the individual TQI steps of "prepare, plan, deploy, and transition." The document became known as the *TQI Implementation Guide;* it was used with awareness training and quality leadership team training at each site and is a valuable addition to the agency's TQI materials.

As we supported the rollout of TQI at the sites in Phase I and II, the master trainers took on the development of additional support documents to respond to facility needs that were not addressed by any external source. The list of documents included the following:

- *Implementation flowcharts:* visual portrayals of TQI implementation from start-up through transition
- *Implementation advisors:* six-page documents highlighting the major components of TQI implementation
- *Implementation checklists:* documents that allowed a medical center to assess its progress in TQI implementation and identify specific activities that could enhance it
- *Education and training assessments:* used to assess training needs, identify responsible staff, plan the delivery of training; and emphasize integration of the TQI education plan into facility-wide education plans
- *Internal consulting skills assessment:* a shorter document than the training manual; given to those throughout a medical center who would be serving in TQI consulting arenas; seen as especially appropriate for physicians championing TQI in clinical areas
- *Awareness booklet:* a short handout that could be given to all medical center employees who attended TQI awareness sessions, to provide them with more information about TQI and a quick reference source

These documents were of high quality, professionally developed and reproduced. Their content was specific to TQI in VHA and, therefore, to health care.

The Rest of the Story

VHA's TQI implementation program was completed in late 1995 with the final training sessions and distributions of funding. The various support activities began to move into the maintenance phase. As we look back, we see an enormous system, national in scope and encompassing widely diverse individuals, cultures, regional differences, and management styles, endorsing and finally embracing a significantly new way of carrying out its business. We now see that the nation's largest integrated health care system is dedicated to the principles of continuous improvement—and this is a federally funded agency. The implications of this course of action are significant, not only for the improvements in health care that will be seen by the veteran patients of the system but also for the likely positive impact those changes will have on all of American health care. There may also be a significant impact on the American medical education system and the federal bureaucracy as a whole. VHA's grand experiment in total quality improvement deserves careful watching over the next few years.

Will the system be able to sustain its initial interest and enthusiasm? A successful implementation of TQI appears to require a certain amount of "front-loading," particularly in terms of a commitment of employee time. But without the opportunities to learn and to adopt new techniques of problem solving offered by TQI, employees will be no better able to cope with the day-to-day situations facing them than they now are. As all of government faces budget restrictions at the end of the twentieth century, such time expenditures may be seen as too expensive or even luxurious. Has VHA been able to train its people well enough already? Are their skills sufficient to not only tackle the issues of the day but also to teach the next generation of workers how to properly address problems "the VHA way"?

Will the press of time and the shortage of resources lead successive waves of managers, supervisors, and employees to revert to previous ways of "solving" problems? Will they once again turn to guesswork and top-down decision making? Will they always settle for just getting the job done? Or have the time, resources, and energy expended in the TQI implementation changed the default mode in VHA employees?

These questions, and many others, will take some time to answer. The initial response of VHA employees to the TQI effort has been highly encouraging; if they are given time and continued encouragement, they likely will show continuous improvement. The results of the team successes outlined in these pages may soon be dwarfed by other, more impressive gains made by the next generation of VHA employees—there are many who are looking forward to that day and planning to collect and circulate those stories and those accomplishments. Perhaps there are two key points to be made about what will be visible in VHA in the future if TQI is a continued success.

First, we should return to the question asked in the first chapter of this book. If VHA has successfully engaged its personnel in continuous improvement, "so what?" What are the gains in patient comfort, improved functioning, or longevity? These are the issues of greatest importance: these are the questions we must answer to convince anyone—including ourselves—that the TQI effort was worthwhile. For clear and obvious reasons, it may be some time before the answers to these questions are evident, longer still before scientific proof is presented. So we may not know right away whether the effort in TQI made by VHA has created clear advantages for its customers, the patients. But we will watch for the answers to these questions, knowing that our final judgment will depend on them. VHA will be collecting the data to address these questions over the next several years.

Lastly, if VHA's efforts are successful in producing salutary improvements in patient care and outcomes, these improvements will come as a direct result of the diligence, perseverance, and thoroughness of the federal employees of the Department of Veterans Affairs. We will know that the time and effort was well spent when we can point to patient-level improvements and know that every VHA employee had a part in producing that success. Such accomplishment may take us to another plateau, where the phrase "good enough for government work" will have regained its original luster and intent: good enough to meet the highest standards known, good enough to be recognized as the best, good enough to be the benchmark.

References

America's best hospitals. (1993, July 12). *U.S. News and World Report*, pp. 66–74.

Berwick, D. M., Godfrey, A. B., & Roessner, J. (1990). *Curing health care: New strategies for quality improvement*. San Francisco: Jossey-Bass.

Quality: How to make it pay. (1994, August 8). *Business Week*, pp. 54–59.The quality imperative. (1991, October 25) [Special issue]. *Business Week.*

Additional Readings

Barnett, T. E., Jr., Ross, S., & Van Dyke, P. (1993). The invaluable team member. *Journal of Healthcare Quarterly, 15,* 22–24.

Batalden, P. B. (1991). Building knowledge for quality improvement in healthcare: An introductory glossary. *Journal of Quality Assurance, 13,* 8–12.

Berwick, D. M. (1989). Continuous improvement as an ideal in health care. *The New England Journal of Medicine, 320,* 53–56.

Berwick, D. M. (1992). The clinical process and the quality process. *Quality Management in Health Care, 1,* 1–8.

Block, P. (1993). *Stewardship.* San Francisco: Berrett-Koehler.

Blumenthal, D. (1993). Total quality management and physicians' clinical decisions. *Journal of the American Medical Association, 269,* 2775–2778.

Brown, M. G., Hitchcock, D. E., & Willard, M. L. (1994). *Why TQM fails and what to do about it.* Burr Ridge, IL: Irwin.

CEO experience: TQM/CQI. (1992, June 5). *The Hospitals,* pp. 24–36.

Crosby, P. B. (1979). *Quality is free: The art of making quality certain.* New York: Penguin Books.

Deming, W. E. (1986). *Out of the crisis.* Cambridge, MA: Massachusetts Institute of Technology, Center for Advanced Engineering Study.

Drucker, P. F. (1974). *Managing in turbulent times.* New York: Harper & Row.

Drucker, P. F. (1980). *Management: Tasks, responsibilities, practices.* New York: HarperCollins.

Fritz, R. (1984). *The pat(h) of least resistance.* New York: Fawcett Columbine.

Geber, B. (1992, August). Can TQM cure health care? *Training,* pp. 25–34.

Juran, J. M. (1964). *Managerial breakthrough.* New York: McGraw-Hill.

Juran, J. M. (Ed.). (1988). *Juran's quality control handbook* (4th ed.). New York: McGraw-Hill.

Kouzes, J. M., & Posner, B. Z. (1987). *The leadership challenge: How to get extraordinary things done in organizations* (1st ed.). San Francisco: Jossey-Bass.

Labovitz, G. H. (1986). *Quality management skills.* Burlington, MA: Organizational Dynamics.

Labovitz, G. H. (1988). *The quality advantage.* Burlington, MA: Organizational Dynamics.

Limerick, D., & Cunnington, B. (1993). *Managing the new organization: A blueprint for networks and strategic alliances.* San Francisco: Jossey-Bass.

Marszalek-Gaucher, E., & Coffey, R. J. (1990). *Transforming healthcare organizations: How to achieve and sustain organizational excellence.* San Francisco: Jossey-Bass.

Maslow, A. H., & Murphy, G. (Eds.). (1954). *Motivation and personality.* New York: Harper & Row.

McGregor, D. (1960). *The human side of enterprise.* New York: McGraw-Hill.

Miller, J. G. (1978). *Living systems.* New York: McGraw-Hill.

Nanus, B. (1992). *Visionary leadership: Creating a compelling sense of direction for your organization.* San Francisco: Jossey-Bass.

Schmidt, W. H., & Finnigan, J. P. (1992). *TQManager: A practical guide for managing in a total quality organization.* San Francisco: Jossey-Bass.

Taylor, F. W. (1915). *The principles of scientific management.* New York: Harper & Row.

Walder, D., Barbour, G., Weeks, H., Duncan, W., & Kaufman, A. (1995, July). VA's external peer review program. *Federal Practitioner,* pp. 31–38.

Walton, M. (1986). *The Deming management method.* New York: Putnam.

Western Region Special Studies Group. (1991, June). *Total quality management bibliography.* Bibliography prepared for the Western Region Managers' TQM Conference, Anaheim, CA.

Wheatley, M. J. (1992). *Leadership and the new science.* San Francisco: Berrett-Koehler.

Index